Conceiving
with *Love*

Conceiving
with *Love*

A WHOLE-BODY APPROACH TO CREATING INTIMACY,

REIGNITING PASSION, AND INCREASING FERTILITY

Denise Wiesner LAc, FABORM

with Linda Sparrowe

Foreword by Randine Lewis

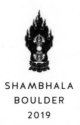

SHAMBHALA
BOULDER
2019

Shambhala Publications, Inc.
4720 Walnut Street
Boulder, CO 80301
www.shambhala.com

9 8 7 6 5 4 3 2 1

First Edition
Printed in the United States of America

♾ This edition is printed on acid-free paper that meets the American National Standards Institute Z39.48 Standard.
♲ This book is printed on 30% postconsumer recycled paper.
For more information please visit www.shambhala.com.
Shambhala Publications is distributed worldwide by Penguin Random House, Inc., and its subsidiaries.

Designed by Allison Meierding

Names: Wiesner, Denise, author. | Sparrowe, Linda, contributor. | Lewis, Randine A., 1960– writer of foreword.
Title: Conceiving with love: a whole-body approach to creating intimacy, reigniting passion, and increasing fertility / Denise Wiesner LAc, FABORM; with Linda Sparrowe; foreword by Randine Lewis.
Description: First edition. | Boulder: Shambhala, 2019. | Includes bibliographical references and index.
Identifiers: LCCN 2018033641 | ISBN 9781611805826 (paperback: alk. paper)
Subjects: LCSH: Conception. | Fertility, Human—Popular works. | Sex instruction.
Classification: LCC RG133 .W54 2019 | DDC 613.9/6—dc23
LC record available at https://lccn.loc.gov/2018033641

I dedicate this book to my late husband, Alex Berks,

who was an amazing writer himself and inspired me with his words.

With our love we conceived our two beautiful children, Noah and Ethan.

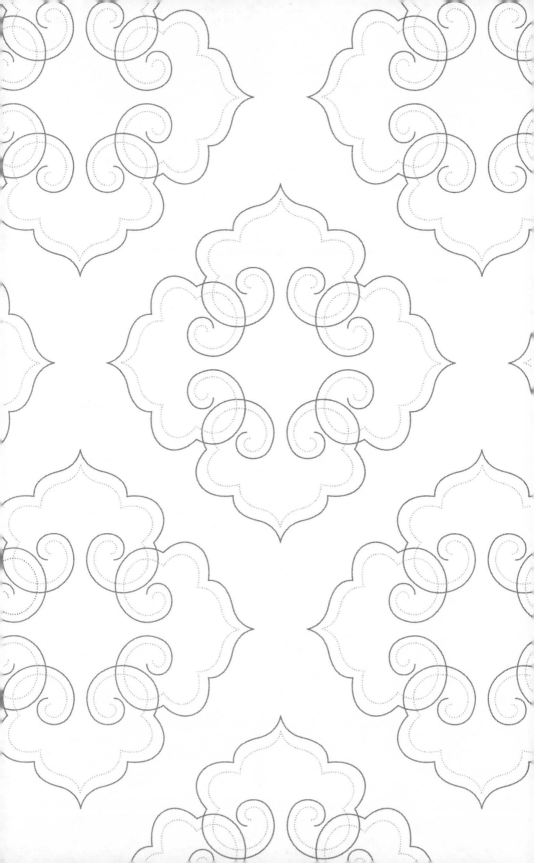

Contents

Foreword

IT IS LOVE THAT CREATES LIFE, and it is love that heals. The radical yet easy-to-follow healing approach of *Conceiving with Love* turns the pain of infertility into the transformative power of love.

The ancient healing tradition of Chinese philosophy recognizes the power of the heart. Our oldest authoritative medical text advises us that the heart is the empress of the body, controlling all of its systems. It is the seat of wisdom, the home of the spirit, and the origin of all transformative healing. When it is deficient or in any way obstructed, all under its domain can suffer the effects of its disturbance. All imbalance ultimately arises from losing connection with the power of our own heart, yet the promise is that all healing comes from the depths within our own heart. I have witnessed this miraculous truth again and again in my own life and in the countless examples of radical healing I have witnessed in those who have come to recognize this same truth. It is the heart that connects us—to our own depths, to others, and to the origin of life. It is through the heart's direct connection with the womb that life is able to manifest.

Imagine a healing process that can improve your fertility, self-awareness, and level of intimacy while experiencing the exquisite pleasure of transformative love. When you begin reading this book, your mind may be occupied with fearful and conflicting thoughts of whether you'll be able to conceive a child. Your journey, like mine, may have taken you through the disillusionment of realizing what conventional medicine has to offer. When these tensions take over your life, it can cut you off from your pleasure centers, your receptivity, and even your ability to heal. By the time you get through this book, Denise Wiesner's labor of love, these thoughts will turn from the stressful mindset of "How can I make a baby?" to "How can I love more deeply?" And believe me, this is the most fertile mindset in existence.

Finally, a conversation about intimacy, sex, and fertility! The sterile procedures of reproductive medicine have little to offer when it comes to ameliorating the sometimes damaging effects that infertility can leave in its wake. Studies have shown that reckoning with infertility can cause the same kind of trauma as that experienced in PTSD—even if you have successfully conceived and given birth previously. Trying to conceive—even naturally, outside of assisted reproductive medicine—tends to turn passion, intimacy, and lovemaking into a cold, goal-oriented pursuit, resulting in frustration and sometimes deep and inconsolable despair. Lovemaking is replaced by mechanical sex commanded by ovulation predictor kits, literally killing our receptivity along with our most important relationships. And yet, as a society, we seem crippled by our reliance on external modalities that falsely offer shortcuts over the true power of inner healing. It seems impossible that surrendering to the heart's ability to experience the depths of intimate pleasure can be the route by which radical healing can occur. And yet, how you make love, how you receive from another and express yourself sexually can reveal what needs to be healed—in your own body, in your feeling center, and in society as a whole. We all have wounds here.

Bringing passion, intimacy, and ecstasy back into baby-making can be the transformative healing power you've been craving. It can truly improve your chances of successfully conceiving and strengthen your most intimate relationship—with yourself. In this way you will transform your outer relationships while creating a blissful, highly energized state into which new life is drawn. Denise dives into the subjects of health, epigenetic inheritance, intimacy, honesty, and trauma during this most important journey toward parenthood—all within the framework of Chinese medicine and backed by science and years of professional experience.

I've known Denise, a dear friend and trusted colleague, for many years. We have shared similar struggles—infertility, heartache, and loss, as well as the transformative healing that Chinese medicine offers. We have each, in our own way, learned to shine within a medical paradigm that simply does not recognize the true power of transformational healing. Like all true healers, Denise has gone into the depths of her own healing process; she has courageously been willing to live as a female warrior and recognize the healing power of love. This is not simply a feel-good self-help book; it is a powerful invitation to break through any barriers that prevent the flame of love and life from burning, to discover what's holding you back from living the most passionate, fulfilling, and fertile life you could possibly imagine.

If you would like to be free enough to be unconditionally happy, ask yourself: Is there enough pleasure, intimacy, love, and gratitude in your life right now? Do you desire to open up your own inner psychic life and experience the courage of sharing the depths of yourself with another? Would you like to experience the transformative power of love as you open up the depths of your soul? It doesn't matter what direction your path is taking you. It may include a completely natural approach or you might involve assisted reproductive procedures. No matter your journey, it is love that opens up the field of miraculous potential through which life arises. We all long for unconditional love. We know its healing potential. You have an opportunity to transcend any lack of love you may be experiencing right now. The love you live will be the greatest offering—to yourself and to your future children.

The undoubtable truth is that life is a miracle, and it cannot be controlled or manipulated into existence. Sometimes we are forced to surrender, to get down on our knees, with nowhere else to turn but to the transformative power of love that lies within the depths of the soul. May this powerful manifestation of Denise's love, brought about through years of her own inner and outer healing work, bring you to the same recognition. It is love that transforms; it is love that heals all; and it is the power of love through which life pours itself into existence.

Randine Lewis, PhD, LAc, FABORM, author of
The Infertility Cure and *The Way of the Fertile Soul*

Introduction

MY OWN ROAD TO MOTHERHOOD wasn't a particularly straight one. At first it was a little too easy, and then it got much harder. I got pregnant right away—six months into a new relationship, in fact. It certainly wasn't how I envisioned the happily-ever-after, you-can-have-it-all philosophy my mother had instilled in me when I was growing up. And to add insult to injury, nine weeks into my pregnancy I discovered that my husband and I were both carriers of Tay-Sachs, a rare genetic disorder. Our baby had a 25 percent chance of being born with the disease, which almost certainly would be fatal. Waiting for the results of the test felt interminable, so when the phone call came with the good news—"The tests came back and your baby is fine"—I cried tears of joy. Nine months later my partner and I were the parents of a beautiful, healthy baby boy.

Three years later, I miscarried, only to get pregnant again three months later—to a Tay-Sachs baby, and sadly we had to terminate the pregnancy at eleven weeks. I spent a lot of time grieving. All I could think about was that second child I so desperately wanted. I checked my cervical mucus, took my basal body temperature, and used ovulation predictor sticks obsessively.

I was so focused on becoming pregnant that all I cared about was getting that sperm inside of me—it didn't matter about the sex part. Once when I was sitting on the toilet I noticed some egg white fertile cervical mucus coming out; I immediately called out to my husband, "Honey, I'm ovulating, let's do it"—hardly a sexy come-on.

For the next twelve months I went to acupuncturists, naturopaths, therapists, and my ob-gyn for help. I was given bags of herbs and supplements. I followed all instructions. All the while I was tired, not sleeping, anxious, sad, bloated, and feeling disconnected from my family and friends. I hated how I felt. I had allergy and asthma attacks. My acupuncturist wanted to treat my lungs, but I didn't care about my lungs, I wanted a baby. I felt sorry for myself. Although my husband was a trooper, neither of us really enjoyed sex anymore; it had become mechanical. There was no intimacy or sensuality; our only goal was to make a baby.

Toward the end of all our struggles, we decided to go away on a vacation with our four-year-old just as I was beginning to ovulate. It was a disaster. We stayed in a yurt with a bathroom outside. A black cat scratched at the screen door all night long. I barely slept. It was summer solstice and a sweat lodge was happening, so we decided to participate. We did all the Native American ceremonies with the group. I prayed to Spirit to put a child in me. When the heavy sweating began, I left the sweat lodge with our son, but my husband stayed. As I was resting, waiting for my husband to return, a woman ran into our yurt and blurted, "Your husband is almost passed out in the tent! Please bring him some water." I ran down the dirt path with a jug of water to the large tent with multicolored yoga blankets on the floor. My husband was sprawled out like a giant sea lion.

"What's going on?" I yelled. "Look what you've done! You've overheated yourself and killed your sperm, and tonight of all nights—I'm ovulating! We're supposed to be making a baby!" He looked up at me, breathing heavily, sipping the water I was trying to pour down his throat. He was so tired he couldn't even speak.

Suddenly it hit me. Had I gone mad? Instead of being concerned about his well-being, I was angry because he was screwing up our chances of having a baby. What was I doing? I stopped and squatted down next to him and reached for his hand. I vowed to regroup and reconnect with the love I felt for my husband. At that moment I realized that babies are made out of love, not desperation. I decided to start counting my blessings and never allow myself to get so far away from what's truly important.

I finally did get pregnant on the fourth try, and now we have two wonderful sons. But I learned a valuable lesson that night. Although by then I had already been treating women with fertility challenges using acupuncture and herbs, my own experience in trying to get pregnant helped me recognize those same feelings of desperation in my patients, whether they were heterosexual or same-sex couples. The women on fertility journeys were suffering, and their partners, suffering in their own way, didn't have a clue as to how to support them. Just like it had been for me and my husband, most of the couples I saw felt that sex had become a chore; urgency and resentment had replaced intimacy and immediacy, and relationships were suffering as a result. The women felt ashamed and alone. As one patient said to me, "We can't really talk to any of our friends—they're either happily pregnant or have kids already."

After hearing these stories over and over again, I began advising couples about subjects too embarrassing for most of them to broach: lubrication, foreplay, positions, orgasm. I felt like my practice had become "sexual confessions in the acupuncture office." I gave my couples homework: exercises taken from qigong, Taoist sexual practices, tantra, Native American intimacy secrets, and plain old common sense. And to their absolute delight, they began having some success. Several conceived naturally, others went the assisted reproductive route, and still others chose to adopt—but almost all of them did so from a place of connection and wholeness. If my patients were starved for this kind of information, I began to wonder how many other people would benefit from it. That's when I decided it was time to write *Conceiving with Love*.

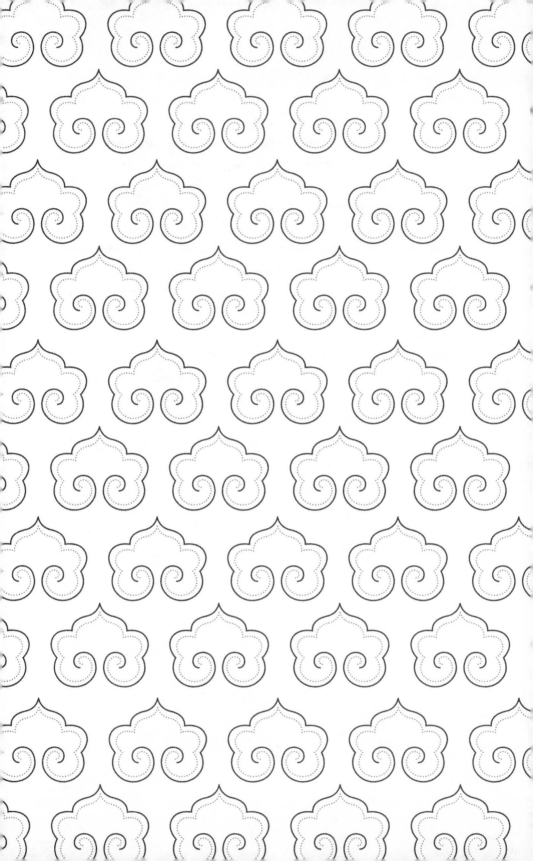

PART ONE

Making Chemistry

1

What's Up Down There?

Knowing others is Wisdom,
Knowing yourself is Enlightenment.

–LAO TZU

THIS MAY FEEL like a return to fifth-grade sex-ed class—for those of you whose school offered it and who weren't too embarrassed to pay attention—but a surprising number of people don't remember exactly how babies are made. I can't tell you how often I've been asked when couples are supposed to have sex, where ejaculate comes from, and whether a woman needs to have an orgasm for pregnancy to occur. I even had to gently remind a few patients of mine that yes, you must have intercourse to make a baby! So . . . let's get started. We'll review both female and male anatomy (external and internal); talk about the importance of the pelvic floor from a Western perspective; and then introduce the energetics of Chinese medicine, where the concept of yin/yang and what's called the "Chinese pattern theory" offer a more poetic approach to the subtler aspects of our physiology. I promise not to make it too much of a snooze.

So, why is knowing your sexual and reproductive anatomy so important? Because by understanding where the pleasure zones are located in your body, you can intensify your connection to yourself and to your partner and thereby maximize your chances of conceiving. By becoming familiar with your sexual anatomy, you'll be able to better guide your partner toward what turns you on and be able to return the favor.

THE FEMALE ROADMAP
External Anatomy

First up, I think it's important to refer to our "private parts" by their real anatomical names. Most women call their genital area their vagina—or any number of silly pet names like pussy, snatch, poontang, cooch, and vajayjay—when what they're really talking about is their vulva. I know, I used to confuse the two myself. But it's the vulva (the jade gate in Chinese medicine, the yoni in Ayurvedic medicine), not the vagina, that contains everything we see when we hold a mirror down there—all the external organs, including the clitoris, two types of labia, the pubic mound, and both the opening of the urethra, so you can pee, and the opening to the vagina. In his book *Petals*, Nick Karras photographed vulvae of all different shapes, sizes, and colors. Like the petals of a flower, each unfolds its secrets to those who have the privilege to see. And the fact is, no two are alike. But how would we even know that? According to research from the Center for Sexual Health Promotion at Indiana University, only 26 percent of women have ever looked closely at their lady bits.

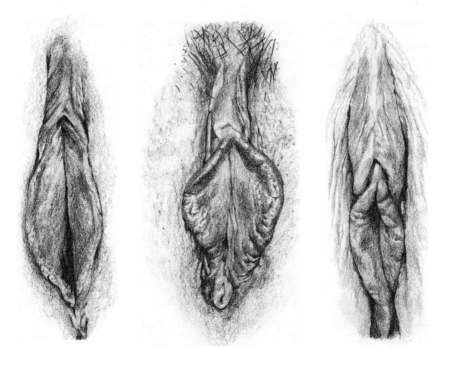

The vagina, on the other hand, is the internal canal, the passageway from the uterus to the vulva through which babies enter the world and a woman's menstrual blood flows. More about that piece of anatomy later.

So why should we say "vulva" instead of "vagina"? For one thing, the vulva is really the sexual pleasure center of a woman's body, not the vagina. Laurie Mintz, author of *The Tired Woman's Guide to Passionate Sex* and a professor of counseling psychology at the University of Florida, intimated in an article that appeared in the *Huffington Post* that by using the term *vagina* to describe their sexual organs, women emphasize the parts of their anatomy that "give heterosexual men the most pleasure"[1] and minimize their own pleasure zones. Using—or at least understanding—the correct anatomical term is empowering. Artist Jacqueline Secor says it so well: "Painting vulvae, focusing on details of women's bodies, even the parts that are 'supposed' to be hidden, does sometimes feel like a small act of resistance—a way of saying that women don't need to hide, that we deserve a place, not just in the art world, but in every sector."[2]

If you're a little reluctant to talk about your vulva, I get it. Call it a vagina, like most of the English-speaking world, if you must. But remember, just the act of naming it without blushing and stammering helps you own your sexuality without shame and gives voice to what you need sexually, without apologizing.

Now that we have the right vocabulary down, let's explore the vulva's various parts in more detail. Feel free to touch your private parts as we go along.

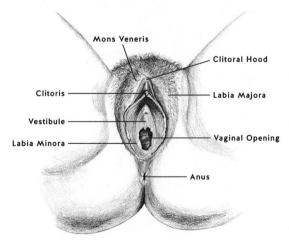

MONS VENERIS: Also called the "pubic mound" and the "mound of Venus," this fatty pad of tissue, generally covered in pubic hair, extends from the pubic bone down to the labia and serves to protect your internal structure from injury.

LABIA MAJORA: These are the outer lips, also covered in pubic hair, formed from the fleshy part of the mons. The size and shape of the outer lips can vary anywhere from 7 to 12 cm. What's the perfect size for you? The one you have! Made from the same embryonic tissue as a male scrotum, the function of the labia majora is to protect the internal genitalia (the labia minora, the clitoris and its hood, and the urethra and vaginal openings). Like the mons, they contain sweat- and oil-secreting glands that produce "pheromones," which are chemicals that are made to impact the behavior of another person. Some say these pheromones are produced by the skin's apocrine and sebaceous glands, which are found in the underarms, the nipples of both sexes, the genitals, the anus, the lips, and the outer rims of the ears.

There's some speculation that pheromones help you attract a mate and increase sexual arousal and may be responsible for syncing a woman's menstrual cycle. This is still a bit controversial because the studies have mostly been done in the animal kingdom. Nonetheless, what a great reason not to cover up your natural scent with perfumes and deodorants, and instead go *au naturel* to the bedroom. One of my patients even said his wife loved to smell his armpits. Case in point.

LABIA MINORA: Surrounded and protected by the labia majora, these hairless inner lips surround the clitoris as well as the openings of the vagina and urethra. They are quite sensitive to touch. Much like their "major" counterparts, their size varies widely—anywhere from 2 to 10 cm. Once again, the size of yours is perfect.

CLITORAL HOOD: Right below the mons, the labia minora connects to form a soft fold of skin, or hood, which hides the tip of the clitoris, called the "glans." If you pull up the hood you will see the glans, the most visible part of the clitoris and, for most women, a highly sensitive spot for sexual stimulation.

CLITORIS: No doubt you already know that this spongy erectile tissue, sometimes called "the pearl," is a pleasure seeker, boasting some eight thousand nerve endings—double that of the penis glans. But did you know that it is comprised of more than just the glans? In fact, it takes up much more vulvar real estate than you think. It has a rubbery, movable shaft—appropriately called the "clitoral shaft"—that eventually elongates, much like a wishbone, into two branches or forks, called the "crura." These extend downward about five inches along the rim of the vaginal opening toward the perineum. Networks of sensitive nerves reach from the crura into the pelvic area. The clitoris is often hidden until it becomes aroused; it then becomes engorged and can deepen in color from pink to burgundy.

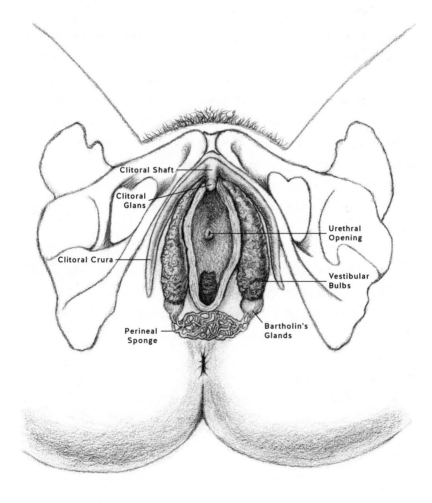

VESTIBULAR BULBS: Also called the "corpus spongiosum," these two bundles of erectile tissue begin where the clitoral shaft and crura meet and continue down the sides of the vestibule, the area that contains the opening to the urethra and the vagina. The vestibular bulbs are on both sides of the urethra and vagina. These bulbs, along with the whole clitoris (glans, shaft, and crura) and the vaginal walls, become firm and engorged with blood during sexual arousal, which produces that urgent desire you may feel to have something put in the vaginal opening and the need to have a release or orgasm.

URETHRAL OPENING: If you take a peek underneath the clitoral hood you'll see a tiny slit right below where the labia minora meets the underside of the clitoris. That's the urethral opening, where you pee. It's the outer part of the urethra, the thin tube that leads to your bladder, which collects urine.

VAGINAL OPENING: The vaginal opening lies just below the urethral opening. At one time this opening was partially covered by your hymen, a thin membrane that (like everything else down there) comes in a variety of shapes and sizes and thicknesses. Some women lose it long before they ever have sex; others feel its demise when they lose their virginity. Although some research suggests that the majority of women don't orgasm with penetration alone, some do experience a sense of fullness that brings them to orgasm.

BARTHOLIN'S GLANDS: Also known as the "greater vestibular glands," these two pea-sized glands that you can't see or feel are located on either side of the vaginal opening. They produce a fluid (mucus) secretion when you become aroused, which makes the opening slippery and wet and easier to penetrate.

Internal Anatomy

Now that we've reviewed our outer anatomy, let's take a peek inside. This is where the actual vagina takes center stage.

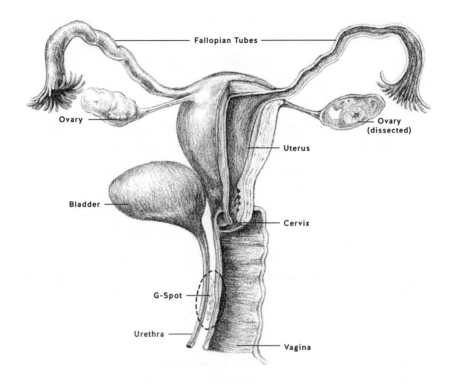

VAGINA: This stretchy, muscular tube, which is the birth canal, contains a network of connective, membranous, erectile tissue that extends from the vaginal opening to the cervix. As I mentioned earlier, this is what connects the uterus and the vulva; it's where your menstrual blood flows and where babies emerge from. You can stick all kinds of things up there—obviously a penis, as well as your finger, sex toys, and tampons.

During arousal, the vagina stretches and can keep lengthening in response to pressure. As you become fully aroused your vagina expands in length and width, and the cervix lifts up as if to welcome penetration—definitely a signal that it's time for intercourse.

The vagina is a complex, dynamic ecosystem mostly inhabited by lactobacilli and bacteroids. Its more than two hundred bacterial species are influenced by genes, ethnic background, environment, and behavior. So treat your vagina with care, which basically means leave it alone. It's self-cleaning, so using soap or douching can mess with its delicate pH.

Glycerine lubricants, which we'll talk about more in chapter 14, can also pose a problem.

G-SPOT: Ah yes, the elusive G-spot, which takes its name from "Gräfenberg spot." First off, scientists are happy to remind us that there's no consensus that a G-spot even exists. But many women would beg to differ. Sometimes called the "urethral sponge," this area is made up of erectile tissue and often has a rough, corduroy texture. Women often report that they experience intense sexual pleasure when the G-spot is stimulated. It's usually found just about two inches inside the front entrance of the vaginal opening, closer to the navel, tucked in back of the pubic bone. Though its exact position varies, it generally appears to encompass the whole length of the urethra, running along the anterior vaginal wall. When a woman gets aroused, this tissue swells with blood, pressing against the urethra (with the help of the pubococcygeus muscle) to keep her from peeing during sex. The structure also includes the Skene's gland, said to be responsible for female ejaculation.

SKENE'S GLANDS: Located around the opening of the urethra, these glands—also known as periurethral or paraurethral glands—may be responsible for the white, viscous secretion thought to be female ejaculation. This ejaculate contains prostate-specific antigen (PSA), which is why the Skene's glands are often called "the female prostate." Don't worry if you can't find these tiny glands or slits; They are nearly impossible to locate unless someone points them out to you. As a gynecologist and sought-after expert on female sexual medicine, Debra Wickman, MD, MS, FACOG, of Banner Good Samaritan Medical Center, in Phoenix, Arizona, theorizes that the Skene's glands of women who ejaculate often becomes more adapted for this function.

PERINEAL SPONGE: Inside the perineum—the area between the vaginal opening and the rectum—lies the perineal sponge. This PS-spot is composed of erectile tissue, which, like the other structures that consist of erectile tissue, becomes engorged with blood during arousal, creating a tighter fit and additional stimulation in intercourse. So as you can see, men aren't the only ones whose sexual organs become erect. Just like the penis, a woman's clitoris, her vestibular bulbs, urethral sponge, and perineal sponge are all made of erectile tissue and become engorged during sexual excitement.

CERVIX: This necklike cylinder, found in the lower part of the uterus, connects the uterus to the vagina. You can feel it easily. Someone once said that it feels like a nose with a dimple in the center. When you menstruate or even during hormonal fluctuations the cervix will change its shape, its position, and even its color. During ovulation it provides a passageway for sperm to move into the uterus through a very small hole (the dimple) in the middle, called the "os." When you're not ovulating, the mucous glands within the cervix secrete an acidic mucus in the vagina, which prevents sperm from surviving. Just before and during ovulation—the fertile window—the mucous glands secrete a more alkaline fluid in the vaginal canal, which is favorable to the survival of sperm.

UTERUS: Called the "sacred cauldron" in Chinese medicine, the uterus or womb is an extraordinary vessel because not only does it discharge menstrual blood, it also holds a baby. No other organ provides such functions. It is composed of three tissue layers: the innermost layer, the endometrium, or uterine lining, where an embryo will implant; the middle layer, or myometrium, composed of smooth muscle; and the outer layer, or serosa. During conception, sperm make their journey from the vagina through the uterus and into the fallopian tubes, where one will fertilize an egg.

FALLOPIAN TUBES: These free-floating tubes provide a special micro-environment for an egg (an ovum), released from the ovary to meet up with some sperm. If sperm are present, fertilization of the egg can occur before it makes its way to the uterus. If not, it'll just move through the tube and be sloughed off as menstrual blood. Small hairlike structures called "cilia" guide the embryo along with a sweeping motion as it grows, until it drops into the uterus around day five or six, and implants around day six to day eight, after ovulation. At the end of the tube are fingerlike projections called "fimbria" that collect the ovulating egg from an ovary each month.

OVARIES: Located on either side of the uterus, these almond-shaped glands are akin to a man's gonads, and they produce follicles that contain eggs. It is said that a woman is born with all the eggs for her lifetime, which are housed on the outer part of each ovary. The ovaries also produce hormones such as estrogen, progesterone, and testosterone.

THE MALE ROADMAP
External Anatomy

When it comes to fertility, men have only one job, albeit an important one: to make a sperm deposit into a woman's vagina, or, if they have opted for reproductive medicine, into a cup. Just like a woman's vulva and vagina, there is no such thing as the perfect size or shape for a man's sexual organs (his penis and scrotum).

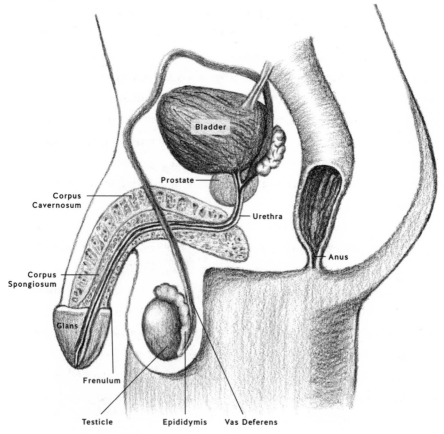

PENIS: No two penises are alike: some are circumcised, some not; some stand straight at attention when erect, others bend like a banana. Some hang to the left, while others prefer the right side—which answers the question tailors often ask, "What side do you dress on?" and prevents them from having an accidental run-in with a penis when they move their hand up a man's leg to measure the inseam.

The average size of an erect male penis is five to seven inches, and the average girth (circumference) is about 4.59 to 4.81 inches. Don't even think about the size of your flaccid penis—it doesn't matter. As one guy told me, "I'm a grower, not a show-er." The penis has three layers of spongy erectile tissue, each of which fills up with blood when the penis gets hard. Some penises grow much bigger when hard; others only slightly. Of course, you can always blame the "shrinkage factor," like George did on *Seinfeld*. In one episode, George has just gotten out of a cold pool when a woman walks in on him naked and laughs at his genitalia. "Obviously," he says later to Jerry, "she doesn't know about the shrinkage factor—you know, what happens to a penis in cold water." Basically, the penis is good for two things: urination and ejaculation—both out of the urethral opening at the head of the penis.

The penis consists of the following parts:

1. **Glans:** Also called the "head" or tip of the penis, the glans is the most sensitive area for most men, especially at the corona, where the head and the shaft connect. This is where the urethra is, the place you pee and ejaculate from.

2. **Shaft:** This tubelike structure extends from the head of the penis to the base, where it connects to your lower belly.

3. **Foreskin:** Unless you've been circumcised, you will have a patch of skin that lies over the glans to protect it. When the penis is erect, the foreskin pulls back to expose the penis tip.

4. **Frenulum:** Another very sensitive spot for a man, this elastic band of tissue is where the foreskin meets the underside of the penis; it is either cut or left intact after a man is circumcised. Dense in nerves, it responds to the squeeze technique when you're trying to control ejaculation (see chapter 5 on edging practice for more details).

5. **Corpus cavernosum:** These two columns of spongy erectile tissue run along the sides of the penis. When more blood fills this tissue than flows out of it, the penis hardens, and voilà, you get an erection.

6. **Corpus spongiosum:** This single column of spongy tissue runs along the front of the penis, surrounding the urethra, all the way to the glans. It also fills with blood during an erection and keeps the urethra open so you can ejaculate.

SCROTUM: Made of smooth muscle and skin and hanging just below the penis, these two sacs are popularly, but not quite accurately, known as "balls." Just like the labia majora in a woman's body, the scrotum's job is to encase and protect the delicate parts of the reproductive organs—in this case, the testicles, nerves, and blood vessels. The scrotum keeps the temperature regulated so that sperm stays viable. If it's too cold, the testicles move closer to the body for warmth; too warm, they move away from the body to cool off. Sexually speaking, many men love their skin on their scrotum tugged. Women should be careful of hitting or twisting the sacs, however—that can be incredibly painful!

Once again, don't worry so much about what your scrotum looks like. Everyone's is different. Most will be wrinkly and hairy, but other than that they can be big or little, symmetrical or lopsided, and can even vary in color.

Internal Anatomy

There are a lot of moving parts in a man's reproductive system. Here's a rundown of the major players:

TESTICLES (TESTES): These two glands, which resemble big olives, are responsible for producing sperm and the hormone testosterone. Unlike a woman, who comes into the world with all the eggs she'll ever produce in her lifetime, a man must "cook up" a new batch of sperm about every seventy-two days. Testosterone is important for maintaining libido, producing sperm, maintaining muscle strength and mass and promoting healthy bone density and healthy vascular function.

VAS DEFERENS AND EPIDIDYMIS: After being made in the testes, sperm accumulate in the coiled tube called the "epididymis," where they can mature and be stored. The vas deferens (Latin for "carrying-away vessel") is a long, thin, yet muscular tube that shepherds sperm from the epididymis to the ejaculatory duct. Secretions from the prostate, which are necessary for sperm survival, as well as secretions from the bulbourethral, or Cowper's gland, mix to form semen. The ejaculatory duct propels the semen into the urethra, where it is carried out of the penis during ejaculation. In a vasectomy, the vas deferens is cut.

PROSTATE: This is a walnut-sized gland located just in front of the rectum, between the bladder and the penis. The urethra runs through the center of the prostate, from the bladder to the penis, letting urine flow out of the body. The prostate secretes a slightly alkaline fluid, milky or white in appearance, which nourishes and protects sperm. During ejaculation, the prostate squeezes this fluid, which makes up approximately 30 percent of the ejaculate, into the urethra, and it's expelled along with sperm as semen.

For some men, massaging the prostate is said to be quite sexually stimulating. In fact, it's often called the "male G-spot." Taoist and tantric sexual practices extol the benefits of massaging the prostate, saying that it does everything from increasing vitality and blood flow to healing trauma. However, if you suspect something unusual is going on, it's wise to get checked out by a health-care professional.

PERINEUM: Located between the anus and the genitals, the male perineum includes the bulb of the penis, root of the scrotum, the penile urethra, the perineal muscles in the urogenital triangle, and the anal triangle. But usually when we speak of the perineum we refer to just the fibromuscular area between the anus and the genitals that can be seen.

From a Chinese medicine perspective, the acupuncture point, Ren 1 (Hui Yin), also called Conception Vessel 1 (CV), is found in the middle of the perineum. Since the nerves in this area can be highly sensitive in some men, I love that Hui Yin is also called Jen-mo, or "million-dollar point." It is the start of the Conception Vessel that goes up the center of the body.

In Taoist sexual practices, pressing vigorously on Hui Yin will prevent ejaculation and instead redirect and reabsorb the activated sexual energy back into the body. Since you are trying to make a baby, you obviously don't want to try that. However, pressing on this point with a *medium* touch sometimes helps a man delay ejaculation and can even increase sensation.

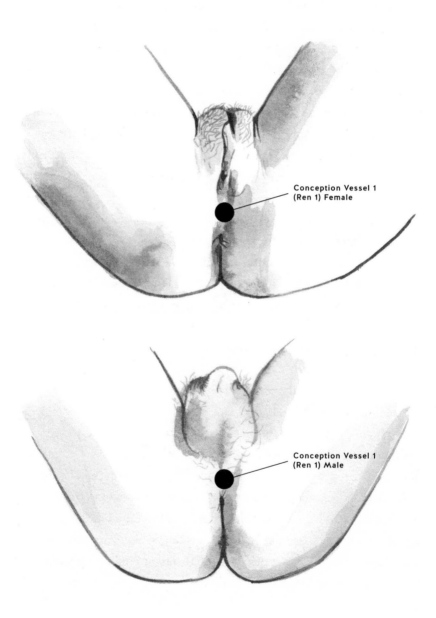

Conception Vessel 1
(Ren 1) Female

Conception Vessel 1
(Ren 1) Male

THE PELVIC FLOOR

Although most people think of the pelvic floor as a "woman's thing," it actually plays an important role in the sexual and fertility health of both sexes. According to Leslie Rickey, a urogynecologist at the Yale School of Medicine, "Pelvic-floor disorders are under-evaluated, underdiagnosed and undertreated in women"[3]—and that's true also in men. Men need to strengthen their pelvic floor as much as women do. Most men just roll their eyes at this suggestion. But a 2008 study published in the *Journal of Sexual Medicine* found that pelvic-floor problems (which include hypertonic pelvic-floor muscles, i.e., muscles that are too tight) contribute to a host of sexual performance problems, including erectile dysfunction and premature ejaculation. If men knew this they'd no doubt be doing pelvic-floor exercises every single day! In fact, aging men who are overweight and who have prostate problems can benefit from strengthening the PC muscle. Research shows that an individualized pelvic-floor muscle-training program can improve erectile function in 75 percent of men. In a small twelve-week study, men were able to help their premature ejaculation by practicing pelvic-floor exercises correctly.[4] Obviously, there are any number of things that contribute to erectile dysfunction, but nonetheless I encourage both my male and female patients to visit a physical therapist who specializes in pelvic-floor dysfunction if they are having issues.

How do you even know where your pelvic-floor muscles are? It helps to think of the pelvis as a hammock or a bowl woven from layers of muscles, ligaments, and connective tissue. Together this structure prevents the contents—all the pelvic organs, including the bladder, intestines, sex organs, and rectum—from spilling out, as well as supports the other organs all the way up to the lower ribs.

Women: You can actually feel your pelvic floor muscles by gently sticking a finger about halfway up your vaginal opening and then gripping it with your vagina. The muscle doing the gripping is the pubococcygeus, or PC muscle, and it controls urine flow, contracts during orgasm, assists in male ejaculation (tell your male partner!), aids in childbirth, and provides core stability.

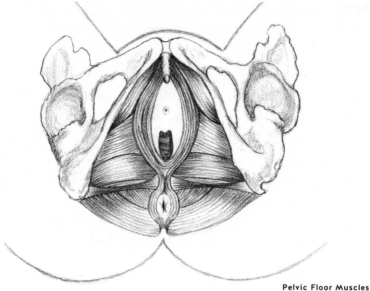

Pelvic Floor Muscles

Men: You guys can tell if you're engaging the right muscles by gently sticking a finger up your rectum and squeezing. Another way is to do the penis waggle. Look in the mirror. If you can move your penis up and down without moving the rest of your body, you've found the right muscle. It's a much better way of discovering and engaging the PC muscle than by stopping the flow of urine.

Kegeling

Kegel exercises can strengthen the PC muscle and can make sex more pleasurable for both sexes. However, it is vital that you fully release the muscle before engaging it again, otherwise you run the risk of overtaxing the PC muscle. Also, men and women don't make a habit of trying to stop the flow of urine—even though that's what some docs will tell you. It's okay to do this when you're first trying to find the PC muscle, but after that, stopping your urine flow is too aggressive a method and can actually weaken it. Instead, gently grip the muscles around your anus (someone said it's kind of like holding those muscles so you don't pass gas in public) and then release completely.

HOW TO KEGEL

1. Sit (with good posture), stand, or lie down (with knees bent and feet flat on floor). Do not tuck your tailbone or suck in your belly.
2. Inhale to release the PC muscle completely.
3. As you exhale, gently draw the muscles up. The operative word here is *gentle*. Kegeling is not about gripping or clenching.
4. Hold the contraction, which involves the muscles in the center of the pelvis, between the vagina (or penis) and the anus for roughly ten seconds.
5. Release the contraction completely for ten to twenty seconds. You should feel all the muscles relax.
6. Repeat the process ten times, as long as you feel the release after the engagement. You can work up to doing one set in the morning, another midday, and a third in the evening if you have a weak pelvic floor.

Pay attention to the rest of your body during Kegels. Do you grip your abs? Your butt? Your jaw? If so, stop. Relax. Start again. Remember: a tense muscle is not necessarily a strong one.

NON-WESTERN ANATOMY

If you're one of the 74 percent of women who have never gotten acquainted with her sexual anatomy, now's a good time to start. Why? According to Amara Charles, an expert in Taoist and shamanic arts and the author of *The Sexual Practices of Quodoushka*, becoming familiar with our own sexual anatomy helps us discover where our erogenous zones are, which in turn will enable us to figure out what type of touch turns us on. As Charles says, "In some anatomy types, the clitoris may be close to the vaginal opening and this will influence how long it will take a woman to reach orgasm. Some women have very little hooding on the head of the clitoris and they barely like any hard pressure there, whereas others, who have long hooding on their clitoris, like a great deal of pressure."[5]

In the Quodoushka tradition, a practice encompassing sacred sexual teachings including practical advice on relationships and intimacy purportedly drawn from ancient Mayan, Olmec, and Toltec cultures, the shape and size of a man's penis can influence the type of arousal, rhythm, and speed that works for him. For example, a "bear man" whose full erection is about one to two hands long and two to four inches thick likes to take things slowly—he'll hug, cuddle, and hold his partner during lovemaking. A deer man, on the other hand, whose fully erect penis is more than two hands and often tapers at the end, prefers prolonged penetration and deep thrusting.

The Kama Sutra is an ancient Indian text on human sexual behavior written by Vātsyāyana around the second century C.E. The Ananga Ranga (Stage of Love) or Kamaledhiplava (Boat in the Sea of Love) is an Indian sex manual written by Kalyanamalla around the fifteenth or sixteenth century. Both of these texts list three types of male and female sex organs based on size. This version of anatomy was used to identify "good fits for good union." These texts also looked at strength of desire and timing to further assess fit.

Three Types of Male Sex Organs (the Lingam)

THE HARE: A man short in stature with a quiet disposition and a moderate sex drive. His erect lingam is not greater than six finger breadths—approximately three to five inches—and his semen usually tastes sweet.

THE BULL: A man with a high forehead, robust stature, and restless temperament, always ready for action in the bedroom. His erect lingam doesn't exceed nine finger breadths—approximately four-and-a-half to seven inches.

THE HORSE: A muscular man with a deep voice, a passionate and reckless nature, and copious salty semen. His erect lingam is about twelve finger breadths—approximately six to ten inches.

Three Types of Female Genitalia (the Yoni)

THE DEER: A woman with a soft, feminine, girlish body, small breasts, solid hips, and an active mind, who delights in the pleasures of lovemaking.

Her vagina cavity does not exceed six finger breadths in depth—about five inches—and her secretions smell like a lotus flower.

THE MARE: A woman with a delicate body and a graceful walk, with broad hips and a long neck. Although she's affectionate, she has a harder time coming to orgasm. Her vagina cavity is nine fingers in depth—about seven inches.

THE ELEPHANT: A large-breasted woman whose feet, arms, and hands are short and fat. Her vagina cavity is about twelve finger breadths—about ten inches—and she has a voracious appetite for sex that is not easily satisfied.

Before you despair that your partner's a Hare and you're an Elephant who really ought to be with a Horse, please remember two things: these anatomical types are generalities that don't take into consideration our complex temperaments, and relationships are much more than what lies below the waist. Also, it's much easier these days to work with what we've got.

Even back in 2598 B.C.E., when Su Nü, a sexual advisor to the Chinese emperor Huang Ti, was asked by the emperor whether the size and shape of a man's penis influenced the "pleasure of communion," she replied, "Differences of size and shape are only external. The true pleasure of sexual communion is based on *internal* feelings. If a man associates union with his partner with love and respect and pure feeling, what could a difference in size and shape do to influence it adversely?"[6]

IT'S ALL ABOUT BALANCE

In Chinese medicine, our health (and by extension, our ability to conceive) depends on our ability to achieve balance—in the body and in daily life. The whole concept of balance takes its cue from the Taoist understanding of yin and yang. Yin energy is feminine in nature—cool, moist, and nourishing; it contains the lunar qualities of stillness, rest, and receptivity. Yang energy, on the other hand, is masculine in nature—warm, transformative, generative; it contains the solar energies of activity, initiation, and doing.

Yin is constant and still, so it makes sense that the eggs in a woman's ovaries lie dormant, resting, since she produces all the eggs she will need for a lifetime at the time of her birth. Yang is ever-changeable, adaptable, so it stands to reason that the testes are busy churning out sperm every single day!

You've no doubt seen the yin/yang symbol, which beautifully reflects that balance. Look closely and you'll notice a dot of yin in yang and a dot of yang in yin, symbolizing the interconnectedness of all things and the coming together of male and female energies. In the teachings of Taoism, making love is a dance of energy. The yin energy of a woman's receptivity meets the yang or fire energy of the man. Conception occurs when yin (egg) and yang (sperm) unite; even lesbian couples who conceive through medical intervention experience this union of yin and yang energies. No matter how a woman conceives, she is at her fullest expression of yin when she is pregnant—even the glow of her skin radiates the abundance of life. Everyone wants to do as much as they can to become pregnant, but the Tao says to find the middle path—both inward and outward. In the I Ching, the yin/yang symbol (*tai qi*) means "you are part of me and I am part of you"; another representation of that symbol looks like this:

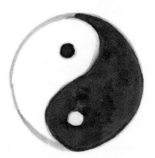

Balance in Chinese Medicine

Chinese medicine's focus is maintaining balance. We must examine the *whole* person and look at all the organ systems, including those of the liver, spleen, lungs, and heart. We assess not only the physical body, but the emotions as well—for example, are you angry, resentful, fearful, or excessively worried? We take into account all the information we can gather, including ancestral information, to form a treatment strategy, which hopefully will increase a woman's ability to conceive.

The Chinese pattern theory says we must keep the body's subtle channels clear in order for qi—vital energy—to flow freely and unencumbered. We must take care to nourish the energy, cultivate it by not going over or under. This means not overdoing things: stressing, worrying, spending, eating, or exercising. It also means not underdoing things either: not giving enough attention to sleep, rest, play, meditation, or connecting with the people we love. The middle path, which is the Tao, keeps us balanced—not too tight, not too loose.

When you are out of balance, you become disconnected from your body and from others, and consequently you may not even notice when your health has become compromised. Stuck qi can contribute to infertility, low libido, and the inability to communicate. The Chinese call this a disconnection between the heart and the loins—fire energy in the heart becoming separated from the fertile water energy in the kidneys. When low fire and water energies combine with stagnation in wood energy (the liver), frustration mounts as pregnancy remains elusive. Metal energy (in the lungs) mixes with an imbalanced earth energy (in the spleen), and grief and worry mount with the realization that pregnancy might never happen. Knowledge of your anatomy and the willingness to listen to your body will help you come back into balance before you get too far removed from your own truth and desires.

How best to do this? Practice wu wei, which literally means "sit still, do nothing." Doing nothing doesn't really mean sitting around all day, doing

> **SEXUAL SECRET**
> *Location, location, location*
>
> Check out your female anatomy. Is your clitoris near your vaginal opening? If so, penetration will stimulate the two simultaneously; if not, you'll want your partner to stimulate your clitoris while you're making love. Many women have a hard time asking for this, especially those who orgasm only through clitoral stimulation. Notice how big your clitoral hood is. Do you have a long hood that covers your clitoris? If so, you might enjoy having it attended to with stroking, fingers sliding all around this covering of the clitoris. If you don't, your clitoris is probably pretty sensitive, so encourage your partner to stroke it more gently.

nothing yet hoping the stork will deliver you a baby. It means living life in harmony with the natural order of the universe, which is the Tao. It doesn't mean you can order up the birth of a child, even if you use Western reproductive medicine. But it does ask you to trust in that natural order even when it feels like nothing is going as planned, even when you fear you'll never conceive.

2

Wet and Hard: The Chemistry and Physiology of Arousal

Your body can stand almost anything.
It's your mind that you have to convince.

–ANONYMOUS

LIKE MOST BODILY FUNCTIONS, what happens "down there" starts with a message from "up here" in the brain, which, if all systems are in sync, will let loose a flood of hormones designed to turn you on. These physiological changes stimulate a variety of erogenous zones—the breasts, G-spot, and clitoris for women; the foreskin and the glans for men; and all the other places that turn you on and increase arousal, passion, and pleasure during sex. Exploring the brain-crotch connection helps demystify how and why we get sexually stimulated; equally important, it illuminates how and why we don't—when men can't get it up and women don't get wet. What happens in the sexual organs when the brain's signals get interrupted because of stress, illness, and other lifestyle challenges? And what can we do to get that connection back in good working order?

Of course, the brain's involvement in sexuality is complex; early experiences and learned behaviors influence how it responds. And since this is not a book on the neuroscience of sex, we'll just stick to the basics in this chapter.

I don't need to tell couples I work with that differences often exist between men and women when it comes to turning up the heat—they tell me! But I do think it's worth exploring why they do and why it matters. Fortunately, there are ancient and modern techniques from a variety of traditions—tantric and chakra practices, for example—that can increase desire for both sexes.

THE SENSES

Sexual desire—the behavioral drive that motivates men and women to fantasize about or seek out sexual activity—can be a powerful motivator, and there's certainly nothing logical about it. Each one of the senses— touch, taste, hearing, sight, and smell—flicks on the desire switch, but the sense of smell is the most notable, particularly when it is triggered by a memory from your past. For example, if your first true love wore a certain aftershave and you walk by someone at a party wearing the same scent, chances are you'll do a double take and will immediately feel a sensation pulsate through your body. If your partner buys the same after-shave, well, that pretty much guarantees your desire to get it on has just increased dramatically. Interestingly enough, it's the *smell* of the after-shave that elicits an arousal response, not a picture of it or a discussion about it.

So why are odors particularly powerful when it comes to memory? One reason is that your body has more than one thousand receptors for odors, which means you can discern among all kinds of smells easily. The other senses don't have nearly as many receptors. Humans also process odors very differently than they do touch, taste, sound, or sight—that is, smells don't go directly to the conscious mind. They first move from the olfac-tory bulb to two parts of the brain: the amygdala, the home of emotional or implicit memory; and the hippocampus, the home of memory creation and recall. The amygdala is not only involved in responding to actual emo-tions (like fear or excitement), but also to *the memory of those emotions*. That means smells are already laced with emotions and memories by the time we are aware of them.

Of course, smell can also be a big turn-on even without harking back to a past event, especially for men. In a study conducted by the Smell and Taste Treatment and Research Foundation of Chicago, researchers found that the smell of pumpkin pie turns men on the most, especially when mixed with the scent of lavender. The investigation determined that 40 percent of subjects were aroused the most by that combination of smells; another 20 percent of the men preferred pumpkin combined with the smell of donuts.[1] That news may entice more women to bake more often and plant lavender! Or, how about some pumpkin-lavender donuts?

A particularly noteworthy study conducted in 2013 at the University of Texas, Austin, and published in *Frontiers in Endocrinology* shows that men can smell a woman ovulating. The study asked 115 men to smell the body odor and genital odor of 45 women. It found that the men's testosterone and cortisol levels increased in response to both odors, but only if those odors came from fertile women around the time of ovulation, and not after it. The subjects hormonal increase apparently lasted longer after smelling the genital odor.[2] And in the now-famous unwashed T-shirt study, males found the odor of ovulating women to be sweeter than the smell of nonovulating women.[3] Who knew? As for women, other studies have noted that we have keener olfactory abilities when we are ovulating; from an evolutionary standpoint, that supposedly helps us choose a mate wisely. Not sure it always works . . .

All this is not to say that the other senses—touch, taste, sight, and hearing—don't play a role in desire or arousal. They absolutely do. Have you ever listened to a song and been instantly transported back to a hot night with a past lover, or cried anew over an old breakup? Accidentally brushed against someone you've been lusting after and felt an electric charge run through your body? Men say all the time that they can simply see a woman and get aroused, and they do—studies bear this out. And I'm here to tell you, so can women! I remember going to a lecture on irritable bowel syndrome—hardly a sexy topic—and being completely mesmerized by the guest speaker, a medical doctor. I've always been a sucker for intellectual men (I guess that makes me a sapiosexual), and this one didn't disappoint. Tall and lean with deep bluish green eyes and salt-and-pepper hair, he had an easy relationship with the material and the audience. Even before he spoke, just watching him approach the lectern I felt my heartbeat quicken, and I began to fantasize what it would feel like to be touched by him. By the time he got to the front of the room, I must admit, I felt more than a little stirring below the waist!

Seeing someone in person is different, however, from seeing erotica on video or reading about it, and studies show that men and women—generally speaking, of course—have different arousal responses to this kind of material. As neuropsychology consultant Carla Clark, PhD, writes in the psychology and psychiatry section she edits for brainblogger.com, "Women are sexually more complex creatures."[4] She reports on a study that showed men responding much more strongly to videos that focused on the physical (sexual intercourse and genitalia predominately), while women prefer videos with a strong emotional component. When women did become aroused watching erotica, they didn't discriminate between heterosexual and homosexual lovemaking—it was all good. Men, on the other hand, only got aroused looking at images of their preferred sex. Of course, measuring women's arousal meter is complex, and trying to do that in a lab setting has its drawbacks for sure.

Although the body doesn't have anywhere near the receptors for touch that it has for smell, touch still plays a very important role in desire and arousal. The theory is that touch—hugging, kissing, holding hands, stroking the skin—releases oxytocin, a hormone masquerading as a neurotransmitter in the brain. Oxytocin is associated with all sorts of positive emotions as well as an increase in empathy, safety, trust, and even generosity and gratitude.

Of course, when we feel good, we get a hit of dopamine from the dopamine reward center in our brain, resulting in a stronger bond of intimacy and closeness; this bond increases sexual receptivity and the longing to be touched, which in turn may increase oxytocin and, once again, may heighten the desire for a repeat performance.

Some studies suggest that oxytocin is higher in people who are falling in love—possibly because they can't keep their hands off each other—and definitely present in both men and women during and after orgasm. It isn't called "the bonding hormone" for nothing. And while couples are busy bonding, their immune systems are benefiting as well. In a 2004 study, researchers found higher levels of immunoglobulin A, an antibody that plays a key role in immune function, in university students who had sex at least one to two times a week.[5] So apparently weekly sex is good for whatever ails us! The wonder of touch is that its benefits are reciprocal. When you hug or massage someone, or take someone's hand, you feel the connection, the bonding, too.

What about food and arousal? I'm not talking about that famous scene in the movie *American Pie*, where Jim, the horny teenager, gets it on with his mother's homemade apple pie. I am talking about our sense of taste— the types of food that turn us on, the act of feeding each other, and even the act of "tasting" each other.

Ancient traditions and modern dietitians champion all sorts of foods— from oysters, pomegranates, and avocados, to Peruvian maca root, Scottish porridge, and dark chocolate—as libido-enhancing. And there are good reasons for this. Many of the touted foods are rich in zinc, essential fatty acids, and other ingredients that increase circulation and optimize the production of sex hormones; others boost energy and desire. And of course the act of feeding each other—whatever foods we choose—is at once intimate and sensual.

At the start of many relationships, the kiss is where we first taste each other. But as we become more intimate, the taste of semen and the taste of pussy become part of the experience. Ideas abound on blogs and websites on how to make our private secretions taste better, including which foods to eat and which ones to avoid. Everyone has a unique taste, and food choices, hormones, and stress levels can alter it. According to Sari Cooper, a therapist, sexologist, and director of the Center for Love and Sex in New York City, "Some people are more sensitive to smell and taste than others. Some men like their partners to go out for a run before they give them oral sex and some like their partners to bathe. There is also flavored lube to help overly sensitive people.... It's all personal preference."[6] Even Napoleon knew this. As the story goes, he was preparing to return home from battle and sent a message to his wife, Josephine, that read: "Coming home in three days: *don't wash.*"

THE STAGES OF SEXUAL RESPONSE

Back in the 1960s, the well-known pioneers of sexual response research, William Masters and Virginia Johnson, popularly known as Masters and Johnson, came up with four stages of human sexual response—excitement, plateau, orgasm, and resolution—that many therapists still use today. A couple gets aroused (foreplay); the excitement builds to a fevered pitch; they both (hopefully) experience orgasmic contractions; and then lie blissfully together in the aftermath, as the sexual organs and the body's systems return to their pre-arousal state.

For many of my patients, especially women, this linear approach to sexual satisfaction can cause a great deal of anxiety and discouragement. First of all, Masters and Johnson's theory presupposes that both partners have to achieve orgasm to achieve satisfaction; secondly, it maintains that both men and women get excited in the same way. What if you *don't* orgasm—a fairly common occurrence in women—and what if you need to be convinced *before* you feel desire? In fact, what if you and your partner have completely different ways of approaching sex?

Luckily, another sexual response model has come along since then that doesn't necessarily negate Masters and Johnson, but rather broadens it. Proposed by Rosemary Basson, a clinical professor at the British Columbia Centre for Sexual Medicine, this model is a bit more cyclical in nature.[7] And while it makes much more sense when applied to women—with a focus on intimacy and the role of desire—I also think it works well for men. Basson believes, as do I, that there is no such thing as a "normal" human sexual response; there is no one way to have meaningful sex. Sometimes a woman's desire comes before arousal; other times being aroused leads to desire. Sometimes both partners climax, or just one, and maybe neither.

Her nonlinear model incorporates intimacy and gives credence to other relationship factors that can affect a couple's ability to have meaningful sex. Couples do much better when they understand each other's needs and ways of responding. I tell my patients: focus on intimacy, learn to communicate, especially to listen to each other, and be patient and generous.

Arousal and Desire

Before we dive into Masters and Johnson's four phases of sexual response, let's take a moment to look at desire. Basson's model suggests that there are two types: spontaneous and responsive. Generally, men enjoy the spontaneous kind, when smelling, seeing, touching, or thinking about someone translates directly into a desire to get it on. So men experience desire first and then arousal. Some women do, too, especially at the beginning of a relationship. But a large percentage of them don't. Their desire is responsive, which means they become aroused by being desired. In other words, arousal first and then the desire for sex. According to Pamela Madsen, a sex and relationship coach, blogger, author, and *Huffington Post* contributor, "For women who have responsive sexual desire . . . it can be really important that they feel sexually desired. If the woman doesn't feel desired, she will probably not be inspired to have sex."[8]

It's also important to note that unlike men, women can be physiologically aroused without physiologically experiencing desire. In other words, a woman may get wet but still not be ready for intercourse—a confusing bit for her partner, who needs to pay attention to other arousal signs such as heavy breathing, moaning, and perhaps rocking of the pelvis. Back in 2004, Meredith Chivers, a leading investigator in female sexuality research at Queens University, Canada, demonstrated that disconnect between physical arousal and psychological arousal.[9] According to Madeleine Castellanos, dubbed "the sex MD," this helps explain why "medications such as Viagra have a significant effect for men, but don't really do much to help a woman's sexual desire,"[10] even though such medications can help fill their erectile tissue with blood.

No matter whether desire comes spontaneously or responsively, what happens in the brain is basically the same for both sexes. Desire and arousal are controlled by the neurotransmitters dopamine and serotonin and the hormone testosterone—in both men's and women's brains. Dopamine controls the brain's reward and pleasure centers and regulates movement and emotional responses. In an article for Harvard University's *Science in the News* titled "Love, Actually: The Science behind Lust, Attraction and Companionship," author Katherine Wu talks about the work of Dr. Helen Fisher, an anthropologist and love expert who teaches at Rutgers University, and she explains that "Lust is driven by testosterone and estrogen, and attraction is related to dopamine along with norepinephrine and serotonin."[11]

The brain's neurotransmitters are so powerful, even in rats. In an old published paper in the '50s by psychologists James Olds and Peter Milner, rats were hooked up to electrodes that stimulated their brains to make dopamine every time they pushed a lever. The researchers found that the rats would keep pushing the lever, even disregarding offers of food, and sex (even though sex does effect dopamine) in order to get a direct dopamine hit (via the brain). Fortunately, as humans we are also wired via the dopamine reward circuit to seek out sex in order to reproduce. I bet you remember when the two of you were so much in love (*and* lust) that being together was all you could think about? That you would have gladly given up food to make love one more time?

When you first see someone who really turns you on, all kinds of things happen in your body and your brain even before you do anything physical. One of the first things your mind does is size the person up sexually and either dismiss them or indulge in an immediate fantasy that quite possibly includes having sex with them. All that noticing and grading their sex appeal happens in the ventromedial prefrontal cortex (vmPFC), which is connected to the limbic system, an ancient part of the brain that drives primal desires, emotions, and memories. No surprise that functional MRI studies show that men have stronger brain activity for visual stimuli than women do, but still, the vmPFC is connected to all five senses, so chances are good that smell, taste, touch, and hearing are stimulated as well.

Next, let's talk about the amygdala. When you see this person who turns you on, this little almond-shaped structure within the limbic system lights up and immediately begins to evaluate and assess the emotional content that you are experiencing and the motivation behind it. Once the person passes that initial evaluation and you're inclined to act, the most active areas of the brain are the anterior cingulate cortex (ACC), known for being involved in pleasure and pain and evaluating risk and reward; the thalamus, which directs sensory information to the proper place; the parietal cortex, which processes and integrates that information; and the hypothalamus, which regulates the release of hormones like dopamine and serotonin. When you begin to feel aroused, dopamine surges, stimulating desire and reward, and you experience a rush of pleasure as the adrenals pump out stress hormones like adrenaline, epinephrine, and norepinephrine, the latter of which can make you feel attracted. You want to pursue that someone! Arthur Aron, a psychology professor at SUNY, Stony Brook, conducted a 1997 study that showed it takes between ninety seconds and four minutes to see if you fancy someone, and body language accounts for more than half of that decision-making. [12] When dopamine levels soar, that lustful connection becomes as pleasurable as the feeling of euphoria that some people feel when they use cocaine or alcohol.

THE EXCITEMENT PHASE: Lots happens in this stage, which involves direct physical stimulation like kissing and petting (or even fantasizing), and it can last for a few minutes or a couple of hours (although the average time for a women to become highly aroused is about twenty minutes). Basically, this is when women get wet and men get hard.

The male sexual response reflects a dynamic balance between the sympathetic and the parasympathetic forces of the autonomic nervous system. When a man is aroused, the parasympathetic pelvic nerves in the penis respond by releasing proerectile neurotransmitters such as nitric oxide and acetylcholine. These chemical messengers signal the smooth muscles of the penile arteries to relax and fill with blood. The veins that would normally drain the blood out squeeze shut, and blood becomes trapped in the penis. This vasocongestion is what creates an erection. The testicles pull in closer to the body, and the scrotum tightens. At this point, some men secrete pre-cum, which is handy for more lubrication.

In a woman, the vagina swells as it lengthens and widens to make room for an engorged penis, as it becomes lubricated with her own fluid secretions. The clitoris enlarges, and in some women the clitoral glans (the knob that we usually define as the clitoris) becomes very sensitive. It retracts under the clitoral hood to avoid direct stimulation from the penis. The labia minora swell and separate, the uterus rises slightly within the pelvis, and the breasts get bigger. All the erectile tissue in a woman—the nipples, vestibular bulbs, clitoris, urethral sponge (the G-spot), and the perineal sponge—engorge with blood, much like the man's penis.

THE PLATEAU PHASE: By now, everything that began in the excitement phase has intensified as the body moves toward orgasm. Breathing becomes more rapid and heart rate and blood pressure continue to increase. Muscle spasms may even begin in the feet, face, and hands.

For men, the plateau phase means the testicles pull up into the scrotum and the urethral sphincter contracts to prevent urine from getting mixed up in the semen. At this point the man experiences a rhythmic pulsation of the muscles at the base of the penis.

For women, what was happening in the excitement phase continues, only with even more intensity. The clitoris becomes extremely sensitive and retreats under the clitoral hood, the Bartholin's glands produce even more lubrication, and the uterus rises up even higher. The vaginal wall turns a darker purple; it continues to swell from increased blood flow, the outer third especially, and the PC muscle contracts to tighten the opening. Breathing gets faster and often more vocalized—moaning and humming—and, of course, heart rate increases as well. Although men can experience flushing of the chest, neck, and face, it more commonly occurs in women. Women may begin to rock their hips and thrust their genitals up and down, in time with their partner's muscular contractions.

At this point, the couple will either climax (the orgasm phase), or if that doesn't happen, move on to the resolution phase.

THE ORGASM PHASE: This is when excitement reaches a feverish pitch and everything literally comes to a climax. For both men and women, energy is released through a series of involuntary muscular contractions. For some women, orgasm can happen when their partner stimulates the clitoris; others prefer pressure on the cervix, the G-spot, or even the perineum, near the anal cavity. As a woman comes, the vagina pulsates, along with the uterus and anal sphincters. According to the 2003 online article, "Biology of Female Sexual Function" appearing in the Boston University School of Medicine, "Orgasm results in repeated one-second motor contractions of the pelvic floor (3-8/orgasm) followed in two to four seconds by repeated uterine and vaginal smooth muscle contraction."[13]

All of this provides intense pleasure, which for some women can last up to several minutes after orgasm. Some women may also feel a shuddering through the whole body; others involuntarily arch their back as they release female ejaculate. This kind of orgasm can also be achieved through masturbation.

For men, usually the orgasm comes first, followed by ejaculation. There is a point of "ejaculatory inevitability"—the point of no return, if you will—where a man can't stop his ejaculation. Like the woman, the man's pelvis may thrust as a series of rapid-fire contractions occurs, which brings extreme pleasure. Generally, the ejaculate comes out in spurts; the first discharge will be the most intense and contains the most sperm.

Physiologically, there's a lot going on while you're getting hot and heavy and about to come. We do know from MRIs that myriad parts of the brain are activated during orgasm. This rather impressive list includes the sensory, motor, reward, frontal cortical, and brain-stem regions (including the nucleus accumbens, insula, anterior cingulate cortex, orbitofrontal cortex, operculum, right angular gyrus, paracentral lobule, cerebellum, hippocampus, amygdala, hypothalamus, ventral tegmental area, and dorsal raphe). Wow!

The sex organs contain thousands of nerve endings, and those nerve endings are connected to three large nerves that travel up the spinal column, plus one wandering nerve, the vagus nerve; all four provide feedback to the brain during sex, which has the brain lighting up all over the place. Luckily, all that feedback is happening courtesy of the autonomic nervous system, which controls all our bodily functions involuntarily. One of these nerves, the hypogastric nerve, communicates between the brain and the uterus and the cervix in women, and the brain and the prostate in men. Another one, the pelvic nerve, focuses on the vagina, cervix, and rectum in women, and the rectum in men. The pudendal nerve shares information from the clitoris in women and the scrotum and penis in men. Just how the vagus nerve participates is not well understood, but scientists do know it transmits information to the brain from the cervix, uterus, and vagina, without going through the spinal cord. All this is to say that if a woman's cervix, vagina, and clitoris are all being stimulated, she could have a pretty intense, very pleasurable orgasm.

Interestingly, the amygdala and the ventromedial prefrontal cortex (vmPFC), both important in regulating sexual behavior and critical thinking, shut down. Scientists speculate that the brain does that so we can suspend inhibition, throw caution to the wind, and reach orgasm.

Do remember that orgasm doesn't necessarily happen every single time you have sex, and that's perfectly fine. In fact, many women report that they've never experienced orgasm with penetration, and yet they still experience satisfaction and plenty of pleasure when making love (see chapter 15 on orgasm for more information.)

THE RESOLUTION PHASE: Once a couple has finished making love and they're wrapped in each other's arms, their muscles begin to relax and the erectile tissue in both partners gradually returns to normal size and position. A woman may still have some vaginal contractions (mini orgasms) as her uterus begins to drop back into place. If she really enjoyed herself, she might be quite happy to go at it again, and her body will oblige, since women don't need any downtime regardless of age. A man, however, has a built-in refractory period that can range from a few minutes (if you're an eighteen-year-old) to fifteen minutes, and for some older men this down-time can last a couple of days, during which time they'll be unable to get it up.

The resolution phase for couples—especially those trying to conceive—should not be cut short. Allow the body and mind to enjoy a postcoital buzz as long as possible, staying high on all those feel-good hormones designed to enhance the possibility of baby-making and keep you healthy. Studies show that oxytocin responds to touch anywhere on the body, and even twenty seconds of sustained hugging will increase that "cuddle hormone."

Of course, all of this happens each time you make love, not just when you first meet someone and sparks start to fly. But nonetheless, there's something quite special about that initial connection. Anthropologist Helen Fisher, who has authored many books on relationships, including *Why We Love*, says, "Romantic love, at its best, is a wonderful addiction." in a 2014 interview with science writer David Levine. Fisher (who is also the brains behind the chemistry.com personality test also used by match.com) says her research demonstrates that "those who had just fallen in love showed activity in regions of the brain associated with anxiety; while with our long-term lovers this anxiety was replaced with activity in brain regions linked to calm and pain suppression."[14] All of this points to how hard it is to return to those lustful, romantic feelings couples had at the beginning of their relationship, especially when various stressors get in the way. But it's worth a try anyway.

ROADBLOCKS TO BABY-MAKING SEX

Now that we have a better understanding of what goes on to produce good, hopefully baby-making sex, let's take a look at a few things that get in the way of pleasure and connection.

We all know the pressure to make a baby can kill arousal for both men and women, but there are many other factors that affect libido.

1. **Stress:** Anytime you're anxious, scared, or stressed, your nervous system is otherwise occupied trying to respond to the danger it perceives. So it automatically shuts down any systems in the body not employed in the act of fighting, fleeing, or freezing—and that includes your reproductive system (more on this in chapter 12).

2. **Medications:** Prescription drugs are often the culprit in squashing a person's sex drive. This includes meds for high blood pressure; antihistamines; birth control pills; pain meds; and antidepressants, especially selective serotonin reuptake inhibitors (SSRIs) (see chapter 15). These drugs not only lower sex drive in both men and women, they can also cause difficulty ejaculating for men and climaxing for women—all of which can put a damper on the desire to get it on.

3. **Fatigue:** When both parties are working all hours and not getting enough sleep, sex drive plummets.

4. **Alcohol:** People often think that drinking loosens inhibitions, and sharing a bottle of wine or downing a couple of cocktails is the perfect antidote to a tumbling sex drive. However, alcohol is a depressant, and we know that depression can cause fatigue and loss of interest in most everything. So it makes sense that overindulging can actually make things worse.

5. **Health problems:** Any urologist will tell you that erectile dysfunction can be a sign of physical and emotional health problems such as heart disease, diabetes, or past traumas. Trauma also prevents women from being able to enjoy sex.

6. **Body issues:** Many women tell me they don't want to have sex because they don't feel good about their body. A positive body image is pretty rare in our society under normal circumstances, but once you add fertility drugs to the equation, things can go negative pretty quickly. Most women who take these drugs say they feel bloated and fat and not at all connected to their body. They don't feel attractive, and the last thing they want is anyone noticing them, let alone touching them. All of this adversely impacts a woman's ability to become aroused. Hormonal fluctuations in both women and men inform their desire— or lack of it. I often recommend that both partners pay a visit to their doctor for some blood work to diagnose any possible problems.

7. **Mismatched lovers:** Yes, indeed, sometimes your lack of desire can stem from being with a partner who's not that good in bed. Face it, your body didn't come with a manual. You learn what you like by touching

yourself and being touched. You learn about sexual positions from books and movies, and in the arms of skillful lovers. Sometimes, asking for what you need sexually—once you figure it out—is the most difficult thing in a relationship. Good communication is one of the secrets of successful relationships, and the topic of sex is no exception.

SEXUAL SECRET

Use these aromatherapy blends to enhance and stimulate passion (courtesy Peter Holmes, founder of Snow Lotus Essential Oils).

For Women

A wonderful aphrodisiac: neroli (bitter orange blossom)
Best all-round oils to nurture her libido: geranium and rose. To use, dilute with jojoba oil and apply to the lower back, sacrum, and lower abdominal area.
Most popular aphrodisiac oils: sandalwood, ylang-ylang, musk seed, jasmine absolute, and tuberose absolute

For Men

Preferred scents: woody aromas such as Atlas cedarwood, Siam wood, sandalwood, vetiver; helps men feel more comfortable with their sexual identity
A special aphrodisiac: a blend of sandalwood, musk seed, and oils with a marine fragrance note such as lavandin, Siberian fir, and celery seed. Holmes says, "The marine note is important because it simulates the odor of human pheromones."

How to use: Use a diffuser to distribute them throughout a room, or add them to your massage oil or to a bath. For women with vaginal dryness, put rose oil in a carrier oil (like jojoba) directly into your vagina.

The Rise and Fall of Passion

For women the best aphrodisiacs are words.
The G-spot is in the ears. He who looks for
it below there is wasting his time.

—ISABEL ALLENDE

WHEN I WAS A LITTLE GIRL, I believed in fairy tales. I couldn't wait to find my own Prince Charming and live happily ever after. I wanted to have it all—a loving relationship, happy children, and a successful career. Of course, the Disney movies back then never talked about what could go wrong with any of this. Everything always worked out perfectly. But over the years I came to understand that the road to happily-ever-after is often a bumpy one, fraught with detours and seeming dead ends, no matter how sophisticated our inner GPS.

So, here's a fairy tale more in keeping with what I witness in my own practice . . .

Once upon a time, in a small mountain town, there lived a married couple, Nicholas and Jennifer. They seemed happy enough, with a cozy two-bedroom house, a golden retriever named Max, and steady jobs—Nicholas as a fireman and Jennifer as a nurse at the local hospital. But truth be told, life had become pretty routine. One summer evening, Nicholas, in his blue and gray flannel shirt and faded Levi's, drove to the market to pick up some fixings for dinner like he did every evening. This time, however, he added a can of shaving cream. It was past time to shave off the scraggly red beard he had grown over the winter and kept in the spring, and anyway he didn't think Jennifer shared his enthusiasm for facial hair. Jennifer worked until eight—her usual shift—so he planned to have dinner waiting for her.

They always sat at the wooden table with its paisley tablecloth, in their yellow-painted kitchen, talking about their day. Jennifer would tell Nicholas about the cases she dealt with at the hospital—on this day it was the eight-year-old boy who broke his leg skiing and an older man who had suffered a heart attack. Nicholas shared his upset at the latest political drama and the details of the day's four-alarm fire. At 10 p.m. they would climb into bed, watch the *Daily Show* with Max sprawled between them, and then drift off to sleep. Many nights Nicholas would wait until Jennifer was softly snoring before going into the other room to pleasure himself.

This particular June night, neither of them could get settled. The full moon's light cracked through the wooden blinds in their bedroom. Finally, Nicholas took Jennifer by the hand and suggested they walk outside. The magic of the night unveiled itself. The sky's darkness was illuminated by millions of stars. They stood side by side on the wooden deck, surrounded by tall, majestic pines and bathed in the gentle glow of the moonlight. After several minutes of silence, Nicholas turned to Jennifer and said, "What's happened to us? What's happened to our love?"

Jennifer didn't answer right away. She ran her fingers through her long brown hair that hung loosely around her gray cotton sleeveless nightgown. She played with the little gold heart around her neck, the one Nicholas had given her just a year ago for their third wedding anniversary—the same week she found out that she had polycystic ovarian syndrome (PCOS) and went off the pill. They had talked about having a baby then, but Jennifer's cycle wasn't regular and she could never predict when she was ovulating. Her gynecologist suggested she try Clomid, a drug to help her ovulate. So for a few months they set their sights on making a baby. Jennifer used ovulation predictor kits; they had sex on demand—but only when Jennifer was ovulating. Clomid didn't agree with Jennifer—she experienced hot flashes and vaginal dryness—so her doctor suggested they do inseminations.

So on top of all the other dos and don'ts, cans and can'ts, Nicholas had to masturbate into a cup on the day of insemination.

After three unsuccessful attempts, they decided to take a break. Unfortunately, so did their sex life. That night in June was the first time either of them broached the subject. After Jennifer failed to respond, Nicholas continued. "We haven't even touched each other since we chose the insemination path. I wanted to give you space because you kept saying you didn't feel sexy. I know you're having a hard time; I know you're depressed. I don't want to pressure you, but I feel so rejected. And so helpless. I don't want to think about making a baby . . . I just want to make love!"

Jennifer started to cry. "I don't need space—I need you! But it's true, going through all that, my body didn't feel like my own. It felt like it had been hijacked by all those fertility hormones. And honestly, I haven't been myself since. Oh Nick, what's wrong with me that I can't make a baby?" By now she was sobbing. "I want to have sex with you, too, but I don't know how to anymore."

The two of them embraced. They stepped back on their path to happily-ever-after that night under the stars, when they agreed to keep communicating honestly and lovingly.

Not all couples are able to talk as openly and tenderly as Nicholas and Jennifer. As a result, they often harbor secret (and erroneous) assumptions about what the other person is feeling and needing. In a 2009 national survey[1] of 259 women and 326 men, 71 percent of women admitted that infertility makes them feel flawed, while 50 percent of men said it made them feel inadequate. But what I find most disturbing is that half of the couples interviewed confessed that they hid their feelings from their partners. When that happens, when couples have no way to process the shame, blame, guilt, anger, or despair they're harboring, those feelings magnify and begin to color everything. Each partner contracts around his or her feelings and is unable to connect with the other. Luckily, there are sex therapists as well as psychotherapists and coaches specializing in fertility who can help couples (or individuals) examine and release their feelings in order to gain perspective and move energy. Helen Adrienne, PhD, author of *On Fertile Ground: Healing Infertility*, says she prefers to work with women individually. "Often the man is the only one she talks to . . . and talks to . . . and talks to. . . . Coming to me on her own is a relief for both of them, and seeing a professional allows her to gain perspective."[2]

Not only do fertility issues prevent couples from being intimate and communicating effectively, they can also cause a rift among friends as well. Women in particular shy away from gatherings with close friends, baby showers, and planned vacations. They especially find it difficult to celebrate someone else's pregnancy. Both partners dread the million-dollar question that friends and family inevitably ask: "So, when are you guys going to have a baby?" They loathe talking about what they see as their failure. With their once-active social life now on hold, couples can become anxious and depressed.

All this is especially true for those using medical interventions. According to a 2004 study, women who visited an assisted reproduction clinic for treatment showed a high incidence of depressive and anxiety disorders.[3] Even back in 1992, Alice Domar, PhD, executive director of the Domar Center for Mind/Body Health at Boston IVF, found that infertile women had twice the prevalence of depressive symptoms as control subjects. I remember talking to a patient of mine who had undergone treatment for a brain tumor ten years prior to her coming to see me. She admitted that the stress of fertility treatments was a lot worse than the stress of having brain cancer. She said that somehow she knew she was going to be okay with the cancer, but she didn't know if she would ever be able to conceive. In fact she now she has two children.

Women aren't the only ones who suffer, of course. In one study, 51 percent of males who had male-factor infertility and chose not to discuss with others the fact that they were going through assisted reproductive technologies (ART) treatment had higher rates of depressive symptoms.[4] It's not the kind of thing that men tell one another over lunch. When asked how their weekend was, chances are slim to none that they'd reply honestly, "Not that good. I tried to have sex with my wife because she was ovulating, but I couldn't get it up. Baby-making sex means pressure to perform, and I failed." All of this produces a vicious cycle: not talking about what they're going through makes men depressed, and being depressed causes a decrease in semen volume and sperm density—which then makes the man feel even more like a failure.

Of course, the problem is that the more a couple obsesses about not conceiving and the more estranged they are from their friends and support group as a result, the more depressed and anxious they become and the less inclined they are to experience passion and spontaneity in their relationship. Studies have shown that infertile couples have significantly higher rates of sexual dysfunction than healthy controls, which is understandable given the pressure to time intercourse and ejaculate at just the right time.

BRING BACK THAT "LOVIN' FEELIN'"

What do passion and spontaneity have to do with making a baby anyway? We all know that babies can be conceived in a petri dish, that a single woman can undergo an IUI (artificial insemination) without even having sex, and that surrogates can carry babies for women who have uterine issues. So since we are quoting song lyrics why not quote Tina Turner, "What's love got to do with it?" Why should we even care about bringing passion back into the equation?

As discussed in chapter 2, from a purely physiological perspective, a lack of passion and focus, especially when laced with anxiety and depression, can adversely impact reproductive health. If either partner is overwhelmed, the chances of feeling amorous, passionate, or even vaguely in the mood can plummet to nonexistent.

What else gets in the way of passion and sensuality? For women, the negative messages we tell ourselves when we're trying (and failing) to conceive are particularly damaging. The body receives these messages (and your doctor's) loud and clear: you are not enough. You are too old, unattractive, and unworthy. The value our society places on what it deems the perfect body—young, skinny, and fit—further sends women who suffer the physical consequences of in vitro fertilization, or IVF, down the I-hate-my-body humiliation spiral.

Janine, one of my longtime patients, perfectly exemplifies what happens when a woman becomes disengaged from her body. She came to see me not long ago, feeling sad and incredibly anxious after a visit to the fertility clinic. The doctor there had told her that her hormone levels were not in the right range so she could not be considered a candidate for Western reproductive medicine at that time. She already knew that her anxiety and the meds she was taking for it were interfering with her sex drive. They were also wreaking havoc on her body, causing her to gain a lot of weight, which further diminished her self-image. In an effort to rein it in, Janine quit her job and began freelancing. Unfortunately, all that time alone fueled her binge eating and self-loathing, which made her feel even worse about her body—and further distancing her from her husband sexually.

Like many women trying and failing to get pregnant, Janine was suffering from a "stagnation of energy," as Chinese medicine puts it. This stuck energy called Liver qi stagnation can block healthy energy flow and disconnects us from our vital, fertile life force, which is also our sexual energy. I began by writing Janine an herbal formula to get the energy flowing again and suggested a meditation and a specific yoga practice to release the tension in her body. As she began to feel better, she lost the desire to binge on junk food and slowly began to regain a little self-confidence. She enjoyed the mirror exercise I suggested (see chapter 8), which helped her relate to her body in a more accepting and loving way. She wasn't so sure at first, when she read the directions, which instructed her to stand naked in front of a full-length mirror and say kind words to her own image, such as "You are strong, you are fertile, you are sexy." But in time she not only became more comfortable naked, she began to notice certain changes in her body that would be beneficial in her quest to become pregnant.

Next on her list: how to reconnect with her husband. After being rejected so many times, he had pretty much given up trying, and the intimacy they once had, which included frequent touching, kissing, and sharing their innermost thoughts, had evaporated. Her husband had put all his energy into his work and was rarely home. With renewed confidence, Janine started by suggesting little things they could do together to show him that she didn't want to be ruled by her hormonal fluctuations and the fear that had consumed her and separated them. Both of them agreed that sex had become associated with failure, and it was time to slowly reclaim the passion they had once felt for each other.

For a man, too, anxiety can play a part in the loss of passion and desire. It often manifests as performance anxiety and fear of failure. When sex becomes mechanical and all about making a baby, both men and women agree that there's nothing sexy about it. When a man feels pressure to perform on demand, when sex can only happen at a certain time (during ovulation), he can sometimes fail to achieve an erection. And if he senses his partner isn't enjoying sex as much as she used to, his self-confidence deflates along with his manhood. David, a patient of mine, confided that he used to love making love to his wife, Lucy. She'd moan ecstatically and routinely have multiple orgasms. But as soon as they started timing intercourse, all that changed. Their lovemaking felt more like an assignment, and soon David was having trouble getting and sustaining an erection. Sex had turned into work, and Lucy, who mourned the fact that she couldn't get pregnant, rejected David's attempts at intimacy at other times during the month. So he stopped trying.

Sometimes a man's passion dissolves because his testosterone decreases (known as "low-T"). This happened to Chloe's husband, Will. When Chloe came to see me about preparing for IVF (although she was thirty-eight, she wasn't quite ready to conceive; she wanted to freeze her embryos for use at a later date), she admitted that her sex drive was much higher than her husband's. It's really not so unusual to have mismatched libidos in a relationship. But as we talked it became clear what was really happening. Will was a hundred-mile marathoner who trained frequently by going on extremely long runs. He also biked long distances. It's been shown that high-endurance athletics such as marathoners, triathletes, and long-distance runners can have reduced baseline androgen hormones (sex hormones such as testosterone).[5] And a 2017 study confirmed that sperm DNA can be affected by high levels of endurance training.[6]

With a little coaching from me, Chloe talked to her husband about his low sex drive and encouraged him to get his hormone levels checked. As a result, he decided to temporarily ease off the training. When he and I met, I recommended a good vitamin supplement and some herbs to replenish his Kidney energy and to help his adrenal glands modulate cortisol. After several months, to their mutual surprise and delight, they were able to get pregnant the old-fashioned way.

Of course, loss of libido doesn't always come as a result of low-T. Having passion in one's life is valuable, but when that passion takes too much time away from a relationship, time together suffers. In our ever-busy society, where people spend most of their day at work or studying (or in David's case, training), fatigue can become a barrier to intimacy. One of my patients said it best: "It's like he's married to his job, not to me."

It's a wonder that we talk about a loss of passion and sexual attraction as if these were essential ingredients for baby-making. Do sparks *really* have to fly in order to conceive? I think the answer is an unequivocal yes-no-maybe. As we saw in our previous examples—David and Lucy, Chloe and Will, and Janine and her husband—rekindling passion can often fast-track pregnancy. It releases tension, anxiety, resentments, and other stumbling blocks and brings couples together in a more loving, less "time-is-of-the-essence" way. Do couples *need* the raging hormones and out-of-control lust they may have once felt when they first got together? No. In fact, for most couples, all that sexual urgency has mellowed by the time they've been together awhile, especially if they're timing intercourse or going through medically assisted fertility. And sometimes the frantic "I can't get enough of you" dopamine-norepinephrine dance can mask other problems in a relation-ship that come screaming to the surface once couples start navigating fertility challenges.

The good news is that such navigation can give couples an opportunity to understand their own conditioning and then create successful strate-gies to overcome their obstacles. You're never too old to learn new ways of being and to see the world with a more tender, open heart. Dr. Joe Dispenza, author of *Breaking the Habit of Being Yourself*, says don't sweat the details: "To experience change: observe a new outcome with a new mind. . . . Hold a clear intention of what you want but leave the 'how' details to the incomprehensible quantum field. . . . To change is to think greater than how we feel."[7] I tell my patients all the time that it's much easier to work on your challenges *before* you've added parenthood to the mix.

THE IMPORTANCE OF GOOD COMMUNICATION

Stan Tatkin, PsyD, MFT, a clinician, researcher, the developer of the psychobiological approach to couple therapy, and the author of *Wired for Love*, believes each of us comes into a relationship with different needs, habits, and ways of relating to conflict. To have a relationship built on love and trust, he says, we must commit to truly listening to and understanding each other's needs. "You are part of a 'couple bubble,'" he says, which means you must put "your partner's well-being, self-esteem and distress relief first," agreeing to take care of each other with devotion and care for yourself as well.[8]

Patience and compassionate communication are especially critical for couples who are using Western reproductive medicine to conceive. Because of the unpredictable effects of fertility hormones, as well as the intense pressure on both partners to perform, couples need to work extra hard in their "couple bubble" to nurture their relationship and revive sensuality. It helps to remember that passion and intimacy aren't limited to—or defined by—how often you have sex.

Approach creating life as a spiritual experience, says psychologist Adam Sheck, known as "the Passion Doctor." Sheck invites couples who come to see him to examine what gets in the way of reigniting the passion they once felt for each other—in the safety of his office. When emotions like anger, sadness, and fear come up, they process those. Sometimes they work on exploring intimacy through physical touch exercises. "I may simply ask them to hug each other, inviting them to explore full body hugs, as though they could melt into one another." The next step, Sheck says, "may be to encourage them to kiss each other—deep, soulful kisses—and explore how that felt: Who gives, who receives, who initiates, where does the masculine or the feminine live in the relationship?"[9]

Not all my patients undergoing infertility treatments struggle in their relationships. One patient, while sporting acupuncture needles in her belly in preparation for a frozen embryo transfer (FET), shared the secrets of her successful marriage: "In the beginning of our infertility journey, my husband had to go through a varicocelectomy [removal of varicose veins in the scrotum]. His doctor gave him supplements to take, but after a month he stopped taking them. He also continued to smoke marijuana even after the doctor told him not to. I was naturally upset but wanted to be strategic about telling him how I felt. I didn't want to attack him. He heard me and made the changes. We've actually gotten closer since doing IVF. One of our other secrets is that we often go away together. We find that staying somewhere other than our bedroom, where we do our fertility injections, is a good way to get back our passion."

Lao Tzu said it best: "Being deeply loved by someone gives you strength, while loving someone deeply gives you courage." I saw the effects of that kind of love one afternoon as I sat with a patient who has type 1 diabetes at her frozen embryo transfer appointment. "I wish I had a clue when we could have sex," she said. "I wish there was more information out there." She and her husband were so in love. I saw the countless ways he cared for her during the time she was in my care, so I just had to ask, "What's the secret to your great relationship?" Covered in a beige heated blanket, lying down on the treatment table at the fertility clinic, she smiled. Her heart was open and her uterus now contained two little grade-A embryos.

"I think it's important to accept your partner for who he is and not try to change him," she said. "It's not as if I can't tell him when he does something that bothers me—I can. But we have great communication. We had to find new ways to be intimate during this fertility process because there were limits on sex. And we did—we do things all the time for each other and we appreciate each other and say so. Like last night, he made me dinner and rubbed my feet."

A constant refrain among those who have been able to hold on to their love for each other and their relationship: embrace the idea of nonattachment and accept things just as they are. Couples struggling to get pregnant get tired of hearing well-meaning friends say, "Just relax and let go. Stop worrying and you'll be fine!" That bit of advice can indeed sound insensitive and callous, but underneath it all lives a kernel of Buddhist truth: We suffer when we become attached to the outcome we desire. We want life to go according to plan. We want people to respond the way we need them to. Truth is, that doesn't always happen. To practice nonattachment, we must accept our beloved fully for who he or she is in each moment, no matter the circumstances. We may want to have a baby more than anything else in the world; we work at it, we do all we can, but ultimately we must let go of trying to control the outcome and trust the natural flow of the universe. Only by living in the moment, honoring all that we feel, and forgiving ourselves and resting in love can we truly arrive in the present.

I shared this Buddhist concept with my patient Linda, who was preparing for her third and final IVF transfer in the hopes of having a second child. She was trying so hard not to be attached to the outcome that she had become anxious and worried. On top of that, she resented her husband for not being as present as she needed him to be. She admitted that she didn't feel like he was taking the fertility process seriously, and that made her angry and sad. "I know his behavior is causing you great suffering," I said to her. "The only way out is to practice forgiveness and nonattachment. That means letting go of how you'd like him to respond and meeting him fully where he is, being present to how he's feeling." She agreed. But I wasn't through: "I also think this holds true for the IVF, Linda. We don't know what the results will be. We'll do all we can and move with love in our hearts. After that, all we can do is trust the journey and accept the outcome."

It is the way of the Tao not to force anything, and that includes sex for baby-making. We must pay attention to the subtle energy of the universe and the go with the flow. For the best outcome, nourish yourself and nurture the exchange between yourself and your partner with heart, spirit, and magnetic attraction.

SEXUAL SECRET

This simple practice can ignite passion without even taking off your clothes.

The Whole-Body Hug

Seems simple, but many couples admit they feel awkward at first. Designed to make you feel safe and loved, this whole-body hug invites you both to embrace and stay awhile. As you settle into the hug, allow your body to melt into your partner's. Feel the rise and fall of your breath against your partner's body and your partner's breath against yours. And then begin to match your partner's breathing so that you are inhaling and exhaling together. Keep surrendering to the experience. If you like, try the whole-body hug naked. Clothed or unclothed, explore this embrace for at least three to five minutes. Hugging activates the parasympathetic (tend-and-befriend) nervous system and boosts oxytocin—the cuddle hormone—both of which promote calm abiding and sweet connection.

What do we need to do to regain connection, intimacy, and passion, especially when things get difficult?

To access our feelings, we need to liberate them first by bringing to light all of our traumas, sorrows, and insecurities—everything that's kept us from acknowledging our passion and celebrating our uniqueness. Once we make space for all that we are, we can more easily treat ourselves with loving-kindness and understand that nothing we feel or think is wrong. I tell my patients and my students to wrap their loving arms around all of their feelings. Everyone thinks *I am the only one who is suffering, the only one with insurmountable difficulties.* But all humans suffer, and yes, all humans are capable of great joy as well.

Love is at the heart of passion, and it is love that creates life. Luckily, there's no age limit or time limit on love and passion. I watched a ninety-second video of an eighty-nine-year-old couple who had known each other since they were ten. "He's always after my body," the woman says happily. "We never carry a grudge and we kiss before we go to bed. We have always held hands. The important thing in a marriage is to be nice to each other and be good friends." Now *that* is passion!

Here are a few ways to reignite the passion between you and your beloved. But don't stop with these—let your imagination run wild!

Use a Talking Stick

This Native American ritual is used to facilitate communication. It's true, a couple can talk and talk and talk, rehashing stories or playing the blame-and-shame game. But often one partner may not feel heard or understood; at other times there's a deeper truth lurking beneath the surface that needs to be looked at. The talking stick gives each partner a turn to express their feelings. It prevents men from jumping in to try to fix things instead of talking about their feelings and women from complaining that they don't feel heard.

BENEFITS: This tried-and-true approach used in group settings is an effective way for couples to practice listening as well as speaking their truth in a way that is kind.

INSTRUCTIONS:

1. Make "I" statements that come from your heart. This prevents you from speaking as a victim, as in: "You never answer the phone when I call so obviously you don't care about me"; or as a persecutor: "You'd better answer the phone when I call"; or as an enabler: "I talked to your secretary, she said you have some time to call me at 11, so I had her pencil it in your schedule." A more authentic way to communicate would be: "I feel sad when I can't get in touch with you."

2. One partner has the stick while the other partner listens without commenting until that person is done speaking. The one listening then reflects back to the speaker what they heard, without stating an opinion. Then they switch places and do the exercise again.

Create Ritual

Years ago, back before cell phones and social media, my husband would light two candles in his room as a sweet invitation for us to switch the energy from the outside world to our inner, more intimate world. It signaled a time dedicated to sexual union, to pleasure, to our life together without distractions. What other rituals can you create with your beloved?

Surprise Date Night

One of my patients came up with this great idea for keeping love energy alive.

BENEFITS: It's playful, spontaneous, funny, and romantic—a bit like courtship, really.

INSTRUCTIONS:

~ One person is in charge of date night one week, and the other person is in charge of date night the next week.

~ When it's your turn for date night, you get to choose anywhere you want to go and anything you want to do. You're under no obligation to share your plans with the other person ahead of time; in fact, it's more fun to keep them on the down-low.

~ On your date night, you are responsible for getting the details together and driving your "date" there. Your date's only job is to show up, be driven to the adventure, and enjoy—in other words, to go along for the ride. This can result in some pretty hysterical evenings.

~ You may pick something that your partner doesn't especially enjoy, and it can even be fun to find out why they don't like it. It can also be enjoyable for your partner to experience something new just because you enjoy it.

HOW WE BROUGHT PASSION BACK

This is the firsthand account of a couple who created a surprise date night to reignite the passion they lost when they were caught up in reproductive hell.

Anyone who knows us as a couple would say we're pretty mushy-in-love. I never understood it when people say marriage is a lot of work, because it feels natural to be close to him. But then we decided to start a family.

There's something quite beautiful about a pregnancy that is the result of love-making between two people who adore each other, and of course that's how we wanted our journey into parenthood to begin. The fact that it took so much effort to become parents—inexplicable infertility and multiple miscarriages—and was fraught with so much pain made us wonder if we were doing something wrong; maybe we weren't trying hard enough or weren't meant to be parents, or (at low points) even meant to be together. It was a very painful period in our life and the result was that it began to erode our friendship and our sense of playfulness, romance, curiosity, and wonder.

Even while we were grieving and unsure about our journey as parents we began doing a few simple things that brought us closer together. Our favorite was date night, done with a couple of fun rules. First off, no dinner-and-a-movie dates. Secondly, it doesn't need to be extravagant, expensive, or even well-planned. If a picnic, a shared bath or shower, or even a walk around the block feels like fun, then do it. Our goal was to get back to the feeling of just being the two of us and being in each other's presence and enjoying each other's company.

There is a practice of surrender, of letting go, of giving and receiving—all important aspects of intimacy. By committing to a weekly date night, we really started having fun again—being playful, romantic, and getting to know more about each other.

For a period of time both my husband and I were extremely busy and didn't have time for our usual weekly date night. We actually needed sleep and rest more than a night out, but we wanted to keep building our intimacy and sense of fun in coming together. So, every night for a month we'd take a walk around the block after dinner for ten minutes, just as the sun was setting. Sometimes we talked, and sometimes we were silent. We would decide what we were open to talking about and what we wanted to bracket for those ten minutes. Some nights we were just silent and held hands. Some of my favorite moments happened during those ten-minute walks.

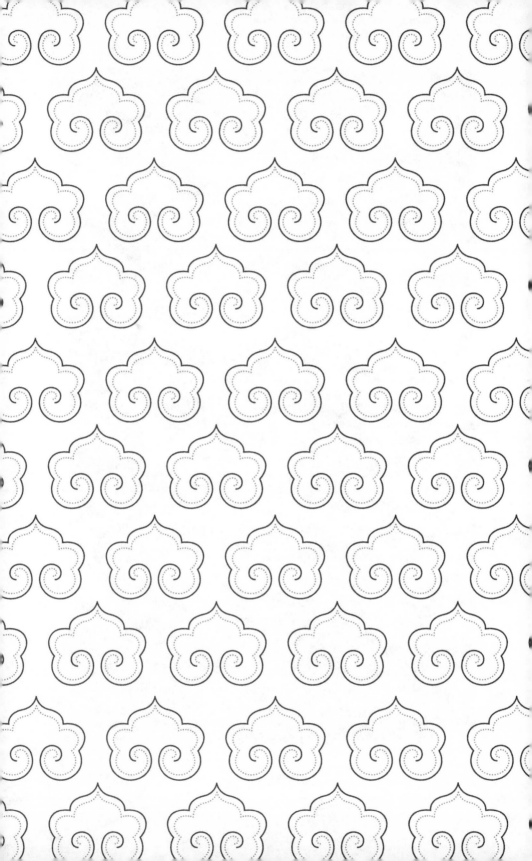

PART TWO

What About Me? What About You?

4

Pleasure Traditions from the East

....

Water is the softest thing, yet it can
penetrate mountains and earth.
This shows clearly the principle
of softness overcoming hardness.

–LAO TZU

I ONCE WENT RIVER RAFTING in Costa Rica with my kids. As soon as you hit a rapid, our guide told us, lean into it. That felt counterintuitive to me—I wanted to push away from it instead. But lean in I did; in fact, I leaned in so much I fell out of my boat. Luckily, it was a shallow part of the river and I was soon reunited with the boat. At the time I thought *What a great metaphor for fertility!* Just like on the river, the challenge is to find the balance between leaning into our experience—not pushing away from everything it brings up, emotionally, physically, and spiritually—and falling into the deep end, where we're unable to get back up and try again. The river element adds to the power of the lean-in metaphor because water, especially in Eastern traditions such as Taoism, tantra, and traditional Chinese medicine, is the primal life force in all living beings. Represented as Kidney energy in Chinese medicine, the water element contains one of the Three Treasures (fundamental energies that maintain human life), known as *jing*. Let's explore what that means and see how these traditions can help us navigate the ever-changing, sometimes choppy waters of baby-making and hopefully give us permission to lean in without drowning.

THE FIRST PRECIOUS TREASURE: JING (ESSENCE)

Jing, usually translated as "essence" or "vitality" in the Taoist tradition, is stored in all living tissue, although the central container and support for jing are the kidneys. Jing presides over growth, maturation, and aging (in other words, all the stages of life). It is your genetic blueprint, and as such it determines pretty much everything about you before you're even born— your physical attributes and your emotional makeup, your strengths and weaknesses, and even who you are on an energetic level. This prenatal jing, located in the lower half of the body, is inherited from your parents; you are born with a finite amount of it and it cannot be replenished. Postnatal jing, on the other hand, can. Think of prenatal jing as our genetic makeup, the energy we acquire from our ancestors. Think of postnatal jing as the energy we acquire out in the world—a combination of epigenetics, the ways in which the expression of our genes can be changed, and lifestyle.

Both types of jing "leak," the ancients say, and those leaks can go at a slow pace or a fast clip, depending on your lifestyle choices. If you've been lucky to enter the world with ample, good-quality jing, and if you treat your pre- and postnatal jing kindly by choosing healthy foods, exercising properly, meditating daily, and taking herbs and supplements, then you have a pretty good chance of slowing your exodus. If, on the other hand, you let your stress levels get out of control—by working way too much, not sleeping, drinking a bit more than you should—you'll deplete your vital essence much faster. The normal wear and tear of living causes jing leaks, as does the aging process, inflammation, and chronic illness, but these other challenges and conditions accelerate the leakage.

Jing is also the generative and creative energy that ensures the viability of the eggs women produce, the health of the uterine lining, and the balance of hormones. In men, jing creates sperm, balances hormones, and enlivens sexual energy. Jane Lyttleton is an acupuncturist, fertility specialist, and founder-director of the Acupuncture Pregnancy and Acupuncture IVF Support clinics in Australia. In her book *Treatment of Infertility with Chinese Medicine*, she says, "jing is translated as 'reproductive essence,'" and goes on to say that "it encompasses the function of the ovaries and some aspects of the pituitary function. Plentiful Jing increases fertility and contributes to longevity."[1]

The quality of a person's jing also determines the body's response to conventional fertility treatments. The stronger the jing, the higher the egg quality and the better the outcome. In Chinese medicine, jing energy governs a woman's menstrual cycle. If she has a weak constitution with a small uterus and intermittent menstrual cycles, we say she has "deficient jing." For men, the quality of jing determines the quality of a man's sperm, his hormones, and his sexual energy. If he has little sexual stamina, poor sperm parameters, and suffers from impotence, then his jing is said to be deficient.

Prenatal jing in Eastern medicine is akin to epigenetics in the West. A 2016 study published in *Biological Psychiatry* showed that the children of Holocaust survivors experienced changes in their DNA. The researchers focused on a particular stress gene linked to PTSD, depression, and mood and anxiety disorders. The results suggest that the Holocaust had an effect on gene expression in people exposed to the horrors of the concentration camps as well as in their offspring, many of whom showed signs of depression and anxiety.[2]

We know that women come into the world possessing a lifetime's supply of eggs, which means you were created from an egg your mother already had when she was a fetus in your grandmother's womb. In other words, your ancestors are intimately involved in your being here. Even if you use a donor egg or donor embryo to have a baby of your own, your blood will interface with the baby's DNA, and that will epigenetically change the way the baby's DNA expresses itself. Research indicates that a pregnant woman's diet can affect her offspring, and that bidirectional cellular exchange between the gestational mother and fetus ensures that the two will stay connected beyond the defined time that the fetus remains in the womb.

So what does all this mean when you're trying to have a baby? First of all, it's important to nourish jing—your vital essence—because it can affect the vitality and health of your offspring. That means you must attend to your emotional, physical, and spiritual health—your inner resources. Otherwise, depleted jing can contribute to a poor response rate to fertility hormones, impotence, and memory decline. In fact, a whole host of factors can adversely or favorably impact a person's epigenetics: diet, seasonal changes, illness, exposure to toxic chemicals, drug abuse, financial status, exercise, prescription drugs, certain herbs and supplements, social interactions, and psychological state.

THE SECOND PRECIOUS TREASURE: QI (ENERGY)

The second of the Three Treasures is *qi* (sometimes spelled *chi*), the circulating life-force energy also known as prana, bioelectric energy, or in the movie *Star Wars*, "the Force." Formed in the middle area of the body, qi circulates via energy pathways called meridians, which loosely correspond to the organ systems in the body. In Chinese medicine we use acupuncture to stimulate qi, which protects the body from external pathogens, regulates temperature, and prevents organ prolapse. Qi helps transform food and air into energy and blood. If your qi is strong, you'll enjoy good health, robust digestion, restful sleep, a balanced immune system, strong and flexible muscles, and a clear mind.

In Chinese medicine, we assess the quality of a person's qi. Low energy, frequent infections, allergies, poor sleep, poor digestion and appetite, depression, poor concentration, and low sex drive are all indications of deficient qi. Excess or pathogenic qi often results when an outside pathogen enters the body such as flu or any number of uterine, bladder, or skin infections. Stagnant qi—energy that's not moving—shows up as frequent sighing, mood swings, distending pain that moves from place to place, irritability, and bloating. PMS is a perfect example of stagnant qi. Luckily, these conditions are treatable using acupuncture and herbal medicine, as well as with diet, exercise, and emotional support.

So how does the quality of your qi affect your ability to conceive? First of all, both women and men need enough good-quality qi for a pregnancy to occur. Women need it during ovulation, for an egg to be released from the follicle, move down the tube to be fertilized, and find its way to its destination. Men need qi for ejaculation to occur. Second, a deficiency of qi means your overall energy will be low and you'd much rather be sleeping than having sex. Stagnant qi can make men and women feel irritable and frustrated, especially when they fail to become pregnant month after month. Third, emotional or physical trauma can cause the qi to get stuck and thus prevent ovulation. And finally, we need qi for an embryo to implant itself in the uterus and a good amount more to hold the pregnancy in place.

THE THIRD PRECIOUS TREASURE: SHEN (SPIRIT)

The last of the Three Treasures is *shen*, which translates all kinds of ways: "spirit," "mind," "consciousness," "God," and "soul"; it can refer to something spiritual, and in its verb form, "to extend." It's often said that jing and qi together provide the foundation for shen.

Shen lives in the upper part of the body, in a person's heart, and an acupuncturist or health practitioner can determine its quality by looking into a person's eyes. Have you ever seen a picture of someone who has committed a heinous crime? Look at the person's eyes—often you'll see a strange or unsettling look about them. This is called "disturbed shen," and it can also happen in cases of severe shock. I once saw this level of disturbance in the eyes of one of my patients whose unborn baby died at thirty-nine weeks because of a cord accident. My heart bled for her, which affected my own shen. According to Giovanni Maciocia, who was a prolific author and practitioner of Chinese medicine, "Emotional life also depends on the Shen of the Heart. With regard to emotions, only the Shen (and therefore the Heart) can recognize them. When we say (or think) "I feel angry" or "I feel sad," who is the "I" that feels angry or sad? It is the Shen of the Heart."[3]

Shen is formed at conception, and according to Lonnie Jarrett, in his book *The Clinical Practice of Chinese Medicine*, shen or spirit is "that aspect of ourselves that is never touched by life . . . and throughout life is always ready to be expressed as absolute virtue the moment we choose to identify with it."[4] In other words, it is our basic goodness, our true essence. When you make love with your beloved and look deeply into your partner's eyes, you connect with their shen. When shen is disturbed, it can dysregulate a woman's menstrual cycle and compromise her ability to ovulate. It can also make it more difficult to sleep and harder for two people to desire each other. Cultivating healthy shen means communicating with love and honesty. It means staying in touch with your own wisdom, your inner knowing. It may mean not rushing into medically assisted reproductive medicine, for example, because your heart tells you to wait a cycle or two. Most important, it means conceiving with love.

The interplay of the three precious treasures, jing (essence), qi (energy), and shen (spirit), is essential for healthy fertility and sexuality. All three areas—the lower, middle, and upper parts of the body—have a continuous energy flow, which enables us to open our hearts to live in love. Strong postnatal jing provides the sperm and eggs with a good hormonal base, but relies on a strong qi to ensure that the right egg and sperm find each other. In turn, this union relies on shen, which is the invisible, infinite energy of love that brings two people together to create life. Even with life's disappointments and challenges, the heart can blossom. This simplified description of the Three Treasures shows the ancient understanding that is still of great value today. The three interdependent treasures are essential for supporting fertility and for enhancing our life force.

YAB-YUM PRACTICE

This classic tantric pose is a wonderful meditation posture for a couple to experience spiritual union. It also prepares a couple for microcosmic orbit breathing (following this exercise, on page 68). In Tibetan tantra, *yab-yum* means "father-mother," or the union of the opposites of yang and yin, compassion and wisdom. In Indian tantra, yab-yum is the spiritual union of Shiva, the male energy, and Shakti, the female energy, with Shakti dancing in Shiva's lap as they gaze into each other's eyes with pure devotion. Some modern tantra practitioners say the union of Shiva and Shakti shows the sacredness of sexuality as a path to the Divine.

1. Have one partner (usually the male in a heterosexual relationship) sit in a comfortable cross-legged position on the floor or on a blanket.
2. Have the other partner (usually the female) sit on the floor, facing her partner. Invite her to straddle her partner, with her legs encircling his waist.
3. Both partners should be equally upright.
4. Spend several minutes in this position, gazing into each other's eyes, touching one another's third eye, or making love.

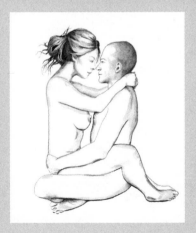

OVARIAN REPRODUCTIVE ENERGY EXERCISE

In Taoist sexual practices, women and men cultivate their sexual energy and then move it to higher centers for physical healing and spiritual awakening. For the purposes of baby-making, we can use this Taoist exercise to awaken sexual energy and connect it to the heart energy and back down to the reproductive organs in order to create life.

Benefits: boosts low libido or flagging sex drive, helps overachievers get out of their heads and into their lower chakras, brings blood flow to the ovaries to tone and support them

Timing: Do this exercise at the completion of menstruation through ovulation.

Instructions:

1. Sit in a chair with your feet touching the floor or stand with your knees slightly bent and connect to the earth energies through the soles of your feet.
2. Place your thumbs together and index fingers together and make a triangle, and place your hands so that the thumbs are resting on your belly button and your other fingers fall close to your ovaries.
3. Make small circles with your fingers, bringing energy to your ovaries as you breathe in and out of the nose with your tongue resting on the roof of your mouth.
4. You can also place a ball or heel of your foot against your clitoris to stimulate it.
5. Now become aware of your PC muscle and begin to draw this energy up nine times. Rest and then repeat two more sets of nine.
6. Move this energy toward the perineum (Ren 1).
7. For more stimulation and arousal of sexual energy, add breast massage (see chapter 5).
8. When enough aroused energy is built up here, use the microcosmic orbit breath (described on page 68) to circulate this energy up

the spine to the brain and down the front line, lingering a bit at the heart space until it is dropped back down to the sexual area. This should arouse a tingling sensation. To enhance this process, choose a nice location, put on some aromatherapy oils, and listen to some sensual music.

SEXUAL SECRET
Increase sexual pleasure by pressing this acupuncture point while making love.

Pressing on the acupressure point Kidney 1 (Yongquan, Bubbling Spring) can enhance pleasure. Kidney 1 (or Kid 1) is located on the bottom of each foot, in a depression about a third of the way down from the second toe, on a line connecting the base of the second and third toes with the heel.

Feet massages are a great tool for foreplay, and if you are massaging your lover's foot, why not place it on your heart chakra (between your nipples)? It's a lovely way to connect the water and fire energies.

For even more pleasure, stimulate Kid 1 while you are making love with your partner. It might require a bit more flexibility and concentration, but it's worth a try. Hint: it works best in the missionary position.

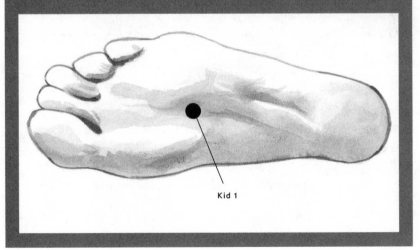

Kid 1

MICROCOSMIC ORBIT BREATHING

Microcosmic orbit breathing, a Taoist practice, is a beautiful way to work with the Three Treasures: jing, qi, and shen. We use the breath to move jing from the lower part of the body up to the middle area where qi is made; and then the two join together, mix with shen at the heart center, and travel back down to the jing level. This circulates the subtle energy, strengthens the hypothalamus/pituitary-ovarian axis, and as a result, awakens your sexuality and fertility. But first, a little background is in order.

Qi circulates in all of our meridians. The two we focus on here are the Ren (Conception Vessel) and the Du (Governing Vessel), both routes for energy to circulate in the body: Ren in the front of the body, and Du in the back. The Ren channel starts by moving qi between the kidneys and then travels up the yin meridians to the depression in the chin, circling the mouth and then entering the eyes. The Du channel also begins at the kidneys but travels up the back of the body, from the tailbone, up the spine, into the brain, around the head, and settling at the upper lip.

These two channels are two parts of the same circuit. Each is connected to the other and together they form a loop of energy that flows throughout the body, connecting yin and yang. Some say this energy loop is like the hypothalamus-pituitary-ovarian axis (HPOA—the three endocrine glands that often act in concert). The qi within the Ren channel controls the birthing process (whether you're giving birth to a child, a creative idea, or a new endeavor) and governs reproductive health in both men and women. It asks the question "Who am I?" The Du channel warms, protects, and ascends energy. We use this pathway for conditions involving the spine or brain; we also use it to nourish our ability to individuate and go forward, seeking independence. Within this channel is the point Du 4, located below the spinous process, the knobby protrusion of the second lumbar vertebra, which is the Gate of Life. This point needs to be stimulated when someone lacks courage, feels timid, or suffers from coldness, weakness, impotence, amenorrhea, depression, or infertility.

We begin by connecting to our sexual energy at the base of the spine and circulating it throughout the body. Basically, what this means is inhaling up the spine and exhaling down the front of the body. Or in Taoist understanding, we charge the energy by moving it up the spine from the lowest chakra to the crown chakra, where the energy of heaven (Du 20) is located; we then bring it back down through the central axis to the heart chakra (Ren 17), and down further into the reproductive organs, thus creating a loop.

Microcosmic Orbit Breathing (Circulating Energy)

1. Sit cross-legged on the floor or in a comfortable position in a chair, with your spine upright.
2. Touch your tongue to the roof of your mouth just behind the teeth to activate the channels. Then begin to scan the body for any tension and release it by taking gentle, full breaths into the belly.
3. Place the palms of your hands on your lower abdomen, with the tips of your thumbs touching directly over your navel and your first fingers touching several inches below your navel to create a triangle shape. This is where your reproductive energy resides.
4. Begin to use abdominal breathing, inhaling and exhaling nine times, to fill the triangle with white light. Breathe gently so that there is no sense of urgency or forcefulness.
5. To charge the energy and circulate it, gently gather this white light and put it in the perineum (Ren 1); inhale it up the spine along the back to the top of the head (Du 20), and then exhale down the front of the body to the genitals, in a circular fashion; do this nine times, gently releasing the PC muscle on the inhalation and slightly engaging it on the exhalation. Once you get the hang of it you can go from nine times to thirty-six, and eventually seventy-two cycles, until you experience a sense of warmth in the belly.

continues

Microcosmic Orbit Breathing (Exchanging Sexual Energy)

1. Sit in the yab-yum position. If this is uncomfortable, simply sit facing each other and hold hands.
2. Begin to practice steps 1 through 5 of the microcosmic orbit breathing, with the exception of step 3. Either continue to hold hands or stay in the yab-yum position.
3. Circulate and build the energy nine times as in step 5 of the previous exercise. When you have circulated back to your Ren 1 (the pelvic floor), in your mind's eye switch your energy to your partner's Ren 1. While maintaining eye contact with each other, create a figure-eight pattern of energy as follows:
   a. Inhaling universal energy from the top of your head, move it down the front of your body to your pelvis and then to your partner's pelvis.
   b. Exhaling, imagine energy going up his or her spine, to the top of his or her head.
   c. Inhaling once again, visualize the energy moving down your partner's center line to his or her pelvis and into yours.
   d. And then finally, exhale it from your pelvis up your spine until it reaches the crown of your head.
   e. Continue moving the energy in this figure-eight pattern nine times. Work up to thirty-six times or even seventy-two cycles.
4. Maintaining eye contact with your partner activates the shen connection.

Don't be concerned if you reverse the inhalation and exhalation; it's moving the energy that counts.

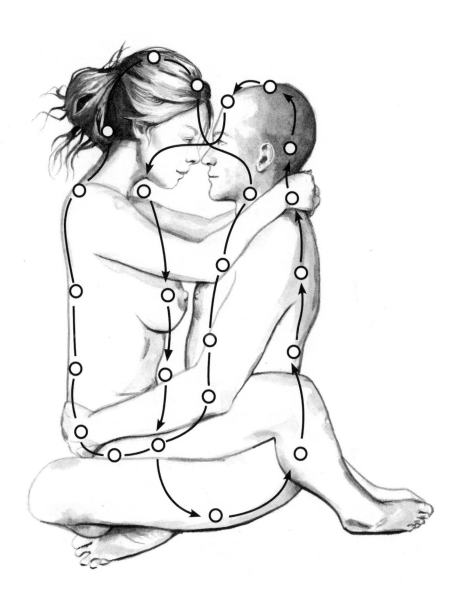

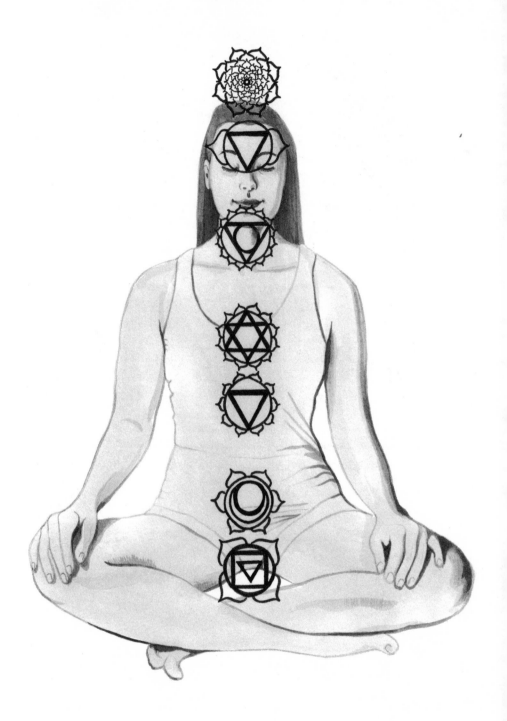

THE CHAKRA SYSTEM OF ENERGY
AND CHAKRA HEALING

So far we've looked at traditional Chinese medicine's understanding of fertility, how important the quality of jing, qi, and shen is, as well as the ability of qi to flow unencumbered through the meridians or energy pathways in the body. We learned that when the flow of energy is blocked, our ability to create life is compromised. The ancient Indian chakra system of energy used in meditation, yoga, and Ayurvedic medicine has a similar understanding of our subtle anatomy. Chakras are wheels of energy that start at the base of the spine and move up through the crown of the head. To elevate spiritually, have more sexual energy, and be balanced in life, yogis say you must clear the pathways, or *nadis*, particularly the central channel, or *sushumna nadi*; this allows the energy to move freely through the chakras. When the chakras are blocked, energy—i.e., life force or prana—can't move and disease (dis-ease) can result.

In the context of this description of sacred anatomy, questions arise. What does your soul need? How can you open up to more love, higher states of being, and spiritual awakening? How can you align these energies with your partner's? How can each of you use these powerful centers to heal your own imbalances and merge your energies? Some say that love relationships work down the chakras: when you first meet, you engage the crown chakra—your energy is electric and ecstatic; moving down into your third eye, your intuition tells you that everything feels exactly right; you learn to communicate, understanding each other's needs and desires using the throat chakra; of course, being in the heart chakra feels effortless, as you bask in the love and connection you feel for each other; the third chakra helps you feel your own power and set boundaries created in love, which opens up the sexual and creative energy of second chakra in the secure, grounded embrace of the first chakra.

Before introducing a chakra healing for couples trying to conceive, I'll give a short rundown on each chakra.

Root Chakra (Muladhara)

LOCATION: base of the spine

FUNCTION: A healthy root chakra connects you to your family of origin, your immediate community, and the global community. The *muladhara* has to do with stability, security, and your basic needs. Through the root chakra you explore your beliefs around sexuality and sexual expression that you've come to embrace from your family and community. This can also manifest in the rules that different religions have about Western reproductive medicine. Sometimes you might find your values are not in alignment with your community's, and you are called to become an explorer of your own truth. The first chakra is where kundalini resides, pictured as a coiled snake at the base of the spine that needs to become awakened.

ELEMENT: earth

COLOR: red

SOUND: LAM

AFFIRMATION: I am safe and connected to source.

Sacral Chakra (Svadhisthana)

LOCATION: between the pubic bone and the navel

FUNCTION: The sacral chakra, *svadhisthana*, is all about relationships, creativity, sexuality, control, money, fertility, and creative expression. When you have a healthy connection with your second chakra you feel pleasure and are able to meet the challenges you face with equanimity. You enjoy your sensuality, and this energy magnifies your intimate moments. Because the second chakra is nurtured by your root chakra, when you feel grounded and supported and loved, chances are your creative expression can flourish. A blocked second chakra, however, can contribute to a sense of rigidity, fear, insecurity, and even, some experts say, to impotence and infertility.

ELEMENT: water

COLOR: orange

SOUND: VAM

AFFIRMATION: I am creative and fertile. I feel pleasure and abundance in every breath I take.

Solar Plexus Chakra (Manipura)

LOCATION: at the solar plexus (the stomach)

FUNCTION: The *manipura* is associated with will and personality; it governs your self-esteem and discipline. A well-balanced third chakra helps people know and live out their life's purpose. Manipura means "lustrous gem," and it is the source of your personal power. When it is balanced, you feel self-confident; you think clearly, make good decisions, and are in tune with your intuition and deeper wisdom. When the third chakra is deficient or blocked you can feel inadequate, irresponsible, or second-guess your decisions. When it's overstimulated you can be manipulative and insist on getting your own way at the expense of others' needs and feelings.

ELEMENT: fire

COLOR: yellow

SOUND: AM

AFFIRMATION: I take care of myself and choose healthy relationships; I love and accept myself.

Heart Chakra (Anahata)

LOCATION: at the center of the chest

FUNCTION: *Anahata*, the heart chakra, is about unconditional love and compassion. This is where yogis say the mind resides—not in the head, but in the heart. A balanced fourth chakra allows us to open more fully to others, giving and receiving with delight. It helps us accept what is, without judgment, and deepens our connection to Earth, to our communities, and to those we love. Anahata is the point in the body where the spiritual energies and earthly energies align and integrate. HazelGrace Yates, PhD, founder of the Cock Project, cuts right to the chase, a man attending her group told me, when she asked him "When was the last time your heart and cock were connected?" When the heart chakra becomes blocked or overactive, you may have a hard time with intimacy and feel disconnected and misunderstood or jealous. Trauma, grief, and loss can contribute to contraction of the heart chakra.

ELEMENT: air

COLOR: green

SOUND: YAM

AFFIRMATION: I am love and I have an abundance of love to give.

Throat Chakra (Vishuddha)

LOCATION: at the center of the neck

FUNCTION: This chakra, *vishuddha*, allows us to speak our highest truth and listen to others without judgment. Your words can have a profound effect on those to whom you are speaking, and the vibration of those words touch your own ears, of course, but they also penetrate your heart. Words can be kind or harmful. Many times couples don't share the same feelings about becoming parents, which makes sharing those feelings difficult and fraught. How can we listen to each other with open hearts? The vishuddha is the source of your truest expression when it is in balance; it puts you in alignment with your higher Self and allows you to speak from the heart. When it's overly stimulated you can talk too much without regard to others, wounding them with your words; it can cause you to be aggressive with your demands and refuse to listen to others. Stagnant fifth-chakra energy blocks your ability to speak, rendering you insecure, timid, and awkward. A balanced vishuddha is essential for couples trying to conceive, helping them to communicate with loving-kindness, understanding, and patience.

ELEMENT: sound

COLOR: blue

SOUND: HAM

AFFIRMATION: I communicate with ease.

Third Eye Chakra (Ajna)

LOCATION: the forehead, between the eyebrows

FUNCTION: The *ajna*, or third-eye chakra, is the center of intuition that allows access to your inner guidance and wisdom. This is where we come to understand that everything is interconnected. Focusing on opening the sixth chakra allows you to gain access to your basic goodness and see more clearly what you know to be true and not succumb to fears and doubts. When the third eye is balanced, you make decisions that move you forward toward your highest good. Acupuncture does this by needling the Yintang point, located approximately between the two eyebrows, at the third eye. When the ajna is out of balance, you may feel stuck in your problems and, lacking clarity or a vision for going forward, see no way out. I often have my patients focus on what it will feel like to hold their newborn baby without focusing on the story of how to make that happen. Seeing their vision becoming reality by connecting to what's true and possible brings calmness to the body and the mind.

ELEMENT: light

COLOR: indigo

SOUND: OM

AFFIRMATION: I trust my inner wisdom to guide me.

Crown Chakra (Sahasrara, or the Thousand Petal Lotus)

LOCATION: the top of the head or slightly above

FUNCTION: This is the chakra of enlightenment and spiritual connection to your higher Self, to all beings, and ultimately to the Divine. It is the center of trust, devotion, inspiration, happiness, and positivity. It also governs your nervous system and endocrine system, the health of which is critical for couples trying to conceive. If the crown chakra is out of balance you may feel isolated, lonely, or disconnected, out of sync with your own body—all of which can happen to couples battling infertility. We need to ground through our roots but also open up to our higher Self to cultivate trust. The seventh chakra receives energy and gives back energy. Life enters from the crown chakra to inhabit the body and life leaves through the crown chakra at the time of death.

ELEMENT: none

COLOR: white

SOUND: OM

AFFIRMATION: I am connected to the wisdom of the universe.

Now that you understand the chakras intellectually, let's discover how they work inside your body to keep you alive, awake, and in balance. The idea is to notice negative experiences and thoughts that you have held in those areas and release and heal them so they can vibrate at a high frequency. Then you will be ready to merge those energies with your beloved—and that's hot!

CHAKRA BALANCING PRACTICE

First, find a comfortable seat on a pillow or lie down on your back. Close your eyes. Take a few deep abdominal breaths through your nose, expanding your belly. Exhale and release any tension you are holding from the day.

1. Bring your awareness down to your root chakra and take a moment to feel the steadiness and stability of the earth beneath you, allowing the earth to hold and support you. Take time now to explore the following: What messages did your family, your religion, or society in general give you about sex and starting a family? Notice any negative messages that come up. How do these messages make you feel? How do they inform the beliefs you hold today? Where in the body do you feel them? On your next inhalation, reconnect with the earth and move the energy into your pelvic floor, at the base of your spine. Inhale through your nose, and as you exhale imagine that those negative messages and beliefs are pouring out from your feet into the earth. Inhale with the mantra, "I am safe and connected to source." Exhale, "I release all negativity."

2. Now, bring your awareness to just below your navel, to the sacral chakra, the heart of your sexuality, creativity, and fertility. Breathe into that space for several breaths and then inquire: *What is in the way of my living fully in my power?* Breathe in the creative life force; exhale out fear and insecurity. Breathing in, "I am creative and fertile. I have pleasure and abundance in every breath I take." Breathing out, "I release all insecurities and doubts."

3. Move your awareness to your stomach, the area between your navel and the top of your rib cage, to your solar plexus chakra. Take several moments to breathe into this chakra and then inquire: *What am I having difficulty digesting? What can't I stomach? How am I caring for myself?* Imagine a yellow light warming your stomach. Breathe the light in and say, "May I be happy"; breathe out, "May I be free from doubt."

4. Bring your awareness to your chest, the home of your heart chakra, and place your hands there. Spend some time breathing in and out of the heart space, releasing any tension or impatience. Picture your partner. Putting aside any frustrations, tension, or sadness that may have entered into your relationship, feel the love you've held in your heart for that person since you've been together. Breathing in, "I open myself up to love," and breathing out, "I forgive you, I forgive myself." Spend some time feeling gratitude for all the challenges you and your partner have faced; see those challenges as more opportunities to practice patience, generosity, and compassion. Remind yourself, "Love resides in my heart. I am love and I have an abundance of love to give."

5. Gently place your hands at the base of your throat, home of your throat chakra. Take several moments to breathe into this chakra, releasing any tension there, and then inquire: *Have I experienced a time when I didn't speak my truth because I was afraid?* Or conversely, *Do I often say what's on my mind without regard for others? Am I afraid of asking my partner for what I want sexually or emotionally?* Keeping your attention on your throat area, visualize the color blue or indigo circulating in and around your throat, thyroid, vocal cords, and esophagus. Tears may come as you release the energy that has been blocking you from expressing your truth. Breathing in, "I speak my truth with clarity and compassion"; breathing out, "I vow to listen with loving attention."

6. Move your awareness to the space between your eyebrows, to the third-eye chakra. Breathe here for several breaths and then inquire: *What is it I truly want? What is our shared vision? What is blocking*

continues

my ability to know? Close your eyes and bring awareness to the center of your eyebrows. Notice what you see there—colors perhaps? Movement within the stillness? Sit with what you're experiencing for a few breaths, and then, breathing in, "I trust my inner wisdom to guide me"; breathing out, "I hold my baby in my arms."

7. Finally, allow your attention to move to the top of your head, to your crown chakra, where we meet the Divine. Take time to simply breathe into this space, visualizing a sense of connection to all that is, a release of all limitations. Breathe in white light from the top of your head and expand your energy beyond your body and out into the world. There is no separation between you and others, between you and the Divine. All things are possible. Breathing in, "I am connected to the magic of the universe"; breathing out, "I release all obstacles to liberation."

5

The Art of Self-Pleasuring

The good thing about masturbation is that
you don't have to dress up for it.
—TRUMAN CAPOTE

ONE COMMON COMPLAINT I HEAR from my female patients trying to conceive is that their sex drive is pretty much nonexistent these days. They're so concerned about timing and the fear of failure that nothing turns them on anymore. Indeed, many women admit that they've forgotten what pleasure feels like, and I'm secretly convinced that some never knew to begin with. When I ask both women and men whether they practice self-pleasuring, many say that they used to, but with the stress of trying to make a baby, hardly ever. My advice? Go back to it. Why? Because self-pleasuring may help women especially get their sexy back. Self-pleasuring allows us to feel sexual excitement without performance anxiety, and that's what we need. In baby-making sex, the goal is to conceive. Nothing else will do. In partnered sex and masturbation, the goal is to orgasm. The simple art of pleasure for its own sake—with or without orgasm—allows us to abandon expectations and be fully present in our bodies, minds, and hearts. And sometimes that's just enough to do the trick.

We all hear reports of people who give up trying, and then they go on vacation, adopt, or just take a break and conceive naturally. I've seen that happen several times in my own practice. Seems too good to be true, doesn't it? But in reality it's not so far out of the realm of possibility. The more we let things be, letting go of expecting a certain outcome, the less stress we feel. Less stress means our nervous system can calm down a lot faster. And less stress often brings positive results. When a woman lets go of goals and expectations, she can focus on pleasure, feeling her own body without the pressure of an outcome or the need to take care of anyone else.

Masturbation, self-love, self-pleasuring—this is a wonderful way to rediscover what gives you pleasure, and then you can share this reawakened sexual energy with your partner. This dance of self-discovery started even before we were children. It began, researchers say, in utero. In 1996 two Italians published a letter in the *American Journal of Obstetrics and Gynecology* reporting that they had observed a female fetus at thirty-two weeks gestation who was "touching the vulva with the fingers of the right hand. The caressing movements were centered primarily on the region of the clitoris."[1] In another paper published in *Prenatal Diagnosis* in 2016, it was found that a thirty-two-week-old male fetus was shown touching himself in utero.[2] Of course, touching genitals in utero is a matter of interpretation, but suffice to say that even infants explore their bodies.

If it helps, the Sexuality Information and Education Council of the United States (SIECUS)—yes, there is such a thing—says that "masturbation is a natural, common, and non-harmful means of experiencing sexual pleasure." That's not all. SIECUS's website also points out that "masturbation can be a way of becoming comfortable with one's body and enjoying one's sexuality, whether or not in a sexual relationship." SIECUS also believes that "no one should be made to feel guilty for choosing or not choosing to masturbate."[3] This is certainly a far cry from the scare tactics your parents no doubt grew up with in the 1950s, '60s, and '70s.

These days it's accepted that children touch their genitals as part of healthy sexual development. According to Dr. Patti Britton, a clinical sexologist and sex educator, "It is our imperative to feel good in our bodies,"[4] and that should happen at a young age. The World Association for Sexual Health agrees: "Sexual health promotion programs . . . should embody the reality that sexual pleasure and intimacy are strong motivating factors for sexual behavior and that sexual pleasure contributes to happiness and well-being."[5] And if all that doesn't convince you, psychologist Noam Shpancer's article in *Psychology Today* should. He writes, "It turns out . . . [that masturbation is a] particularly important predictor of sexual health and happiness for women, more so than for men. One of the best predictors of whether a woman will be able to achieve orgasm in her sexual relations is a history of masturbation in adolescence."[6]

I could go on and on citing statistics—there are so many—but I won't. Suffice to say, if you do love to self-pleasure, you're in the majority, and as we know, majority rules! According to a 2016 report, 89 percent of women and 95 percent of men admit to masturbating; 40 percent of men masturbate daily, 22 percent of women masturbate daily, and 53 percent of women use vibrators to self-pleasure.

As for me, I never got up close and personal with my vulva until my late forties, but I certainly know how to self-pleasure and have been doing that ever since I was a little girl. I remember one nap time in kindergarten when I got restless and began to touch myself over my cotton underwear and pleated wool skirt while facedown on my stomach, trying to relax. My teacher came up to me and with a firm voice said, "Denise, it's not okay to do that here." I felt so ashamed that I never told anyone, not even my parents, what had happened. Early messages like that carry on into adulthood and color our feelings about self-touch. I wondered how many other men and women had a defining moment like mine that reinforced our culture's taboo around masturbation. The answer has revealed itself through my patients.

THE MANY BENEFITS OF SELF-PLEASURING

Bella came to me after being diagnosed with lichen sclerosus, a condition affecting the vulva that caused the eroding of her labia and the hood of her clitoris. The shame Bella felt around having a "disfigured" vulva made her not want anyone to touch her, and she certainly didn't want to go there herself. Bella assured me that this condition was rare—and embarrassing. I assured her it was more common than she realized, though rarely admitted or discussed. I went on to say that many of us have a complicated relationship with our "private parts" and that she was definitely not alone.

"Thanks," she said, "It's true. I didn't even know what mine looked like." I didn't either, I told her; in fact most women don't. When I asked about her upbringing, she said she was raised Catholic, and there was a great deal of shame when it came to sexuality. She ended up "acting out as a teenager," which caused more shame and guilt.

Boom, I got it! On an unconscious level, Bella had internalized the notion that having sexual feelings was "bad" and that lichen sclerosus is divine retribution for experimenting sexually and even enjoying it. Yet Bella was ready to reclaim her right to sexual self-pleasure. To that end she embarked on a treatment plan that combined acupuncture and Chinese herbs to reset her immune system with body-based therapy to heal the trauma surrounding her shame and guilt. She was amazed that her lichen sclerosus diminished, along with her self-incrimination.

So why focus on masturbation—a decidedly solo endeavor—in a book for couples wanting to create more intimacy and enhance fertility? For several reasons. First of all, talking about sex with the person you love is critical to creating a more loving, sensual connection. On the other hand, not talking about your sexual needs—especially when you're in baby-making sex mode—can cause friction and make you feel alone and frustrated. The problem is that women often don't know what they like, and men are too embarrassed to ask for what they want. So how the hell can you possibly convey your needs to your partner? Luckily, playing with yourself can help you figure out what turns you on, which can then lead to honest, nonjudgmental communication.

Case in point: A patient of mine—I'll call her Jasmine—and her husband, Blake, were having difficulties conceiving. She was frustrated because Blake couldn't seem to get it up during her fertile window. He, on the other hand, was terrified of being a father, which certainly messed with his sexual prowess. Turns out that the thought of having a baby brought up his trauma around his father walking out when Blake was five years old. He began therapy to heal old wounds and to give him the tools he needed to be able to share his concerns and fears with Jasmine. He got enough nerve up to tell her he didn't want to know when she was ovulating; he just wanted to have more regular sex. During the time that Blake was having his difficulties, Jasmine took to self-pleasuring, where she discovered that she needed much more clitoral stimulation before she could climax. She found she liked her clitoris gently stroked in the beginning and then a firmer, consistent side-to-side motion after that. She also found her G-spot with a special sex toy and enjoyed having it stimulated along with her clitoris. She decided to show her husband how to use his fingers as foreplay on her clitoris and G-spot to bring her to orgasm even before he put his penis inside of her. Doing that also aroused Blake. Being able to talk about what they each needed and what gave them pleasure brought them closer together. They began to have more pleasurable intercourse and more often, and six months later Jasmine got pregnant.

Self-pleasure, according to Planned Parenthood, has many benefits, including fourteen mentioned on its website, plannedparenthood.org. Some of my favorites, especially with regard to sexuality and baby-making, include increasing well-being, enhancing the sexual experience both physically and emotionally, improving your relationship with your partner, creating a more loving connection to your own body, learning how you like to be touched sexually, having more orgasms, stress relief, and increasing self-esteem.

Taking the time to discover what makes us feel good is the ultimate in self-care. As women, we are responsible for our own orgasms. And since research says that most women orgasm with clitoral stimulation, wouldn't it be helpful to find out how your vulva and vagina would like to be caressed?

But exactly how should you go about doing all this? Is there a right way and a wrong way to masturbate? Generally speaking, slow down! Most people learn to do it quickly, eager to get to orgasm or fearful of being walked in on. There is a sexual practice known as "edging," which allows a person to delay orgasm. According to the International Society for Sexual Medicine, "Some people find that this technique makes their orgasm more intense, once it does occur."[7] When a man practices edging it can help him delay orgasm so he can be more in sync with his partner. Women who use this technique say it helps them turn localized orgasms into whole-body orgasms. What edging means for a man: bringing yourself just to the brink of orgasm, stopping, starting again, stopping. Working up to twenty minutes of this, according to the experts at *Cosmopolitan* (and other sexologists), will make you a pretty awesome partner.[8]

When I was doing research into self-pleasuring, my inquiry led me to an interesting video on the subject, in which a dark-haired female in her forties used the Magic Wand, a high-powered vibrator, on her clitoris. I know it sounds pornographic, but really it was more of a tutorial on specific techniques women and men can use to pleasure themselves—alone and with each other. I learned so much! I wanted to watch it because there's so much confusion, and a bit of controversy, surrounding vibrators. Some people fear that using vibrators desensitizes a woman's clitoris and makes her less responsive to human touch. Others think that if a woman needs a vibrator on her clitoris, in addition to penetration, then her man is inadequate as a lover. None of this is true. Sure, you may have heard stories about women who have basically jackhammered their clitoris for years and can't seem to orgasm with their fingers, but that's not the norm.

So, here's where the Chinese medicine principle of balance comes into play. If you have become accustomed to only using a vibrator to orgasm, try changing things up. Experiment with your fingers, which may bring erotic sensations you've not experienced before. Bring sex toys to your solo practice, as well as to your couples practice, and see what happens. Make sure to reinforce the idea that the toy is not a substitute for your partner's tongue, penis, or hands. Toys are an every-now-and-then enhancement; don't let them detract from the love that is exchanged during lovemaking. (For more on toys, see chapter 14.)

A SOLO PRACTICE FOR WOMEN

1. Bring a towel and lubricant (like coconut oil) to a special area you've set up. If you've chosen a bed, dress it with sensuous sheets and beautiful pillows. Include other items—erotic books, movies, candles, and music—anything that brings in sexy.
2. Lie on your back and notice your breath. Gently encourage your breathing to be smooth and long.

3. Using the breath, begin to bring energy into your yoni. As you inhale, squeeze the vagina, rock the pelvis forward into a pelvic tilt, and gently draw the energy up to the cervix. Then, as you exhale, bring the energy back to your perineum as you release the pelvic tilt and slightly arch your back. Do this until you feel warmth in your yoni.

4. Softly brush your legs, inner thighs, arms, and abdomen with your hands, feeling the texture of your skin. Become aware of sensations.

5. Now touch your breasts, your nipples. Practice using different pressures—light, pulling, pinching—to feel what gives you pleasure.

6. Put your hand over your mons and send loving awareness to this area. Rotate the palm of your hand in a circular motion and notice how that feels. Thank your reproductive organs for their capacity to bring forth life.

7. Work your way down to your clitoris, placing your fingers around the hood, using gentle pressure. Maybe use a little coconut oil for lubrication. Arousal makes it possible to touch your clitoris directly, but first just touch the clitoral hood. See what feels good. Rock your pelvis back and forth.

8. Breathe, move, make sounds. Sound frees energy and lets us be in the moment. According to tantra and Taoist teachers alike, making sounds opens the throat chakra.

9. When you feel aroused, pull the hood of the clitoris back to expose the glans so that you can try different ways of touching your clitoris. Gently touch it with the pad of your index finger. Add more fingers. See how that feels. Stroke the clit with the pad of your finger downward lightly, just like you would touch your eyelid. Try it at the one o'clock position on the left side of the clitoris with a very light up-and-down stroke. As arousal magnifies, try rubbing it back and forth and side-to-side; notice the effects of the different speeds, pressures, and sensations. You get the idea. Explore! Have fun!

10. Rub the vestibular bulbs on the inside of the inner labia and see how that feels. There's erectile tissue there, too.

11. Lastly, you might feel the urge to put something into your vagina to experience a sense of containment. Use your fingers to explore your vagina and feel the texture there. Can you find your G-spot, located on the anterior wall of the vagina? Sometimes it helps to push out your vagina to expose it. Try rubbing it or giving it pulsing pressure. You can also use a toy—they make ones especially for G-spot stimulation. You can even stimulate your clitoris with one hand and your G-spot with another.

12. Orgasm not required, but if one or even multiple ones happen, wonderful!

13. Lastly make sure to *love* your body as is. It is your temple; it is life-giving; it is perfect.

What about men? Dr. Philip Werthman, an authority on male infertility and a reproductive urologist at the Center for Male Reproductive Medicine and Vasectomy Reversal in Los Angeles, says that during the fertile window men should refrain from masturbating and "should be having sex with their partners," unless, of course, they have to leave their deposit in a cup for an insemination or an IVF.[9] Beyond that, masturbation can certainly be a great way for a man to learn how to delay his orgasm if he's an early ejaculator. (As well, see the instructions for the edging practice later in this chapter.)

Of course, reasons for ejaculation issues such as early and delayed ejaculation are varied and complex. According to a study published in the journal *Translational Andrology and Urology*, "a single pathogenetic pathway does not exist for sexual disorders generally." In fact, a variety of biological, psychosocial, behavioral, and cultural factors contribute to "trigger, reinforce, or worsen the probability of DE (delayed ejaculation) occurring."[10] These include high blood pressure, antidepressants (especially SSRIs), intimacy issues and performance anxiety (both comon during fertility challenges), ambivalence about having a baby, and anger or resentment toward your partner.

Even though masturbation can help some of these challenges—it's cheap and easy—it can also exacerbate intimacy problems. Men who have been masturbating since early boyhood may have gotten into the habit of quick release to avoid being found out. Others may have a vigorous masturbation style, which is so unlike the stimulation they experience during penetration that they have a hard time ejaculating during lovemaking. Obviously, if you or your partner are experiencing some of these issues, you'll want to consult with a urologist to rule out medical problems.

My male patients often tell me they feel the pressure to "make" a baby, pressure to get it up, and pressure to come on demand—all ingredients in a surefire recipe for an erection fizzle. What's a guy to do? First and foremost, breathe. All Eastern traditions use the breath as a way to calm the nervous system. In this case, a few rounds of conscious breathing can get you out of your thinking, judging, reactive mind and into your body so you can simply feel the sensations that come up.

Try the self-pleasuring (and mutual pleasuring) techniques below. If nothing helps, consider going to a sex therapist who can help you deal with the complex underlying factors that are preventing you from baby-making.

FOR MEN: EDGING PRACTICE FOR EARLY EJACULATORS

This solo practice teaches a man how to delay ejaculation in order to spend more time pleasing his partner.

1. When you self-pleasure, notice your point of no return, when ejaculation is inevitable. Pay attention to body signs and sensations such as heavier breathing, sweating, and pelvic rocking.
2. Once you know the signs of impending orgasm, stop all self-touching and practice conscious breathing until the urge to ejaculate has passed.
3. Other ways to stop ejaculating include breathing and tightening the PC muscle (although some men find relaxing the PC muscle works better), pressing the "million-dollar point" on the perineum with your second and third finger (the Chinese pressure point called Ren 1), or simply squeezing the base of your penis with your hands (squeezing technique).
4. Once you gain control of your arousal and ejaculation, you can practice with a partner. When you feel like you're about to come when you're inside your partner, stop all movement, practice conscious breathing, tighten the PC muscle, or squeeze the base of the penis—the remedies listed above.

Note: If you have delayed ejaculation or can't ejaculate into your partner because of what's called an "idiosyncratic masturbatory style"—in other words, your style of masturbation provides different friction than your partner's vagina—then you should discontinue masturbation or alter your style. Some sex therapists advocate using the other, nondominant, hand to masturbate in such cases.

SELF-PLEASURING TOGETHER

Self-pleasuring doesn't need to be a solo sport. One way to explore each other while eliminating the pressure to perform is through "sensate focusing," a four-part practice that Masters and Johnson introduced. In the first stage, a couple touches each other everywhere except the erogenous zones (such as the genitals and breasts), without climaxing. The focus is on sensual experiences and a mindful investigation of each other's bodies. This can take the pressure off performing and get both partners back to touching each other for pleasure. (More on this in chapter 13.)

The next step after sensate focusing is to set a self-pleasure "date," in which one partner watches the other pleasing him- or herself. This can be a total turn-on. Add music, sensual fabrics, sexy lingerie, candles—basically anything that gets you in the mood. If your date happens during the fertile window, use this as a foreplay technique; if not, let the volcano erupt.

Most people would agree that self-pleasuring can be an intimacy enhancer, but not everyone would say the same about pornography, especially the kind men use to "get in, get off, and get out." The internet, of course, makes it easy to find all kinds of pornography and a vast array of erotica. What's the difference between the two? The most common understanding is that pornography depicts sexual behavior, the sole intention of which is to arouse to climax; erotica, which aims to celebrate the human form through art, literature, or film, has a more aesthetic sensuality and sensibility to it. Leon Seltzer, PhD, a psychotherapist, author and blogger for *Psychology Today*, believes that porn is "cheapening—for *both* sexes—the whole experience of physical intimacy" and is merely an outlet for "alleviating stress or sexual tension." Erotica, on the other hand, aspires "to celebrate the varieties of sexual bliss and the universal desire for carnal union," he says.[11] Jumping on the anti-porn bandwagon, psychiatrist and psychoanalyst Norman Doidge, MD, in his book *The Brain That Changes Itself*, says that when his patients stopped using pornography, they were able to reverse impotence and sexual arousal problems, and feminist author and journalist Naomi Wolf, in her book *Vagina*, believes that, "chronic masturbation to porn sexually desensitizes men overall."[12]

SEXUAL SECRET
A Taoist Technique to Awaken Sexual Energy in the Ovaries

What do Taoists say can help a woman become aroused? Breast massage—done either alone or with a partner. Taoists believe that the breasts awaken the sexual energy in the ovaries. In tantra, the breasts, as the gateway to the genitals, are said to stoke the Shakti fire. The breasts are how we nourish life, and between them is the anahata, the heart chakra, the center of love. Massaging your breasts every day increases circulation and helps eliminate stagnant energy, which can help prevent disease in the breast. To gain the greatest benefit from this self-healing massage, practice every day—from a few minutes to fifteen minutes. Attending to your love and sensuality can result in some delicious sensations.

1. Find a comfortable seated position, using pillows to prop up your hips if necessary. To increase arousal, sit so that the heel of your left foot rests on your vulva. If this is too difficult, take a ball and place it between your heel and vulva. Begin by taking nine full breaths, inhaling and exhaling through the nose.
2. Rub your hands together vigorously with some oil to warm the energy. Use coconut or almond oil and, if you wish, add a few drops of essential oil. Nadine Artemis, creator of Living Libations, shares her special blend of breast massage oil in her book *Renegade Beauty: Reveal and Revive Your Natural Radiance*. It's a therapeutic massage oil containing 55 ml jojoba oil as a carrier oil, to which you add 5 ml orange essential oil, 10 drops laurel essential oil, and 10 drops frankincense essential oil.
3. Place your whole hands on your breasts, close your eyes, and pause, taking three deep breaths, dedicating your massage to self-love. Use an affirmation such as "I embody love" if you wish.
4. Start with the palms of your hands covering your nipples; move your hands around your breasts in an outward direction, with a gentle but firm pressure. This is the "dispersing energy"—moving the right hand in a counterclockwise direction and the left hand clockwise about twelve times. Now massage your breasts in an inward direction—this is the "condensing energy."
5. Next, using your fingertips, massage the area about an inch and a half around your nipples, which activates the endocrine glands, including the pineal, pituitary, thyroid, and the adrenals, as well as the ovaries.
6. To increase arousal and sexual energy, continue to massage your breasts until you feel energy in your yoni. For added stimulation, inhale and hold your breath and then squeeze your nipples as you pump the PC muscle ten times, then exhale. Repeat this twelve times.

Many people don't agree that porn itself is the problem. Marty Klein in his 2016 book *His Porn, Her Pain* says, "The ultimate issue in many couples in conflict about pornography is the decline or disappearance of their once-enjoyable sex life. This is extremely hard for couples to discuss, given the shame, grief, confusion, rejection, failure, and hopelessness that people often feel." He also adds, "a lot of porn use is actually a desperate attempt to stay in a sexually unfulfilling couple. If couples could talk about sex honestly and directly, most antagonistic conversations about pornography would just go away."[13] I agree with him that the issue isn't porn—it's that we don't know how to talk about sex in the real world.

Regardless of how we define erotica or judge porn, some couples actually find watching porn together to be a real turn-on, a way to liven up their sex life with a bit of novelty, which enhances the brain's dopamine reward circuit. Soft porn, created by women for women, has proliferated online—from films with a sensual storyline around a real love relationship to short takes showing sex-positive attitudes and displaying all different kinds of real bodies to tutorials on how to masturbate. Clearly, there's something for everyone these days. And if you're not into the visuals, amazon.com has more than sixty thousand titles under the banner "erotica by women." You're welcome.

Self-pleasuring is a way to increase self-love. Don't be afraid to experiment. Don't be afraid to be a sexual explorer, an adventurer. Sexuality is part of our birthright as women and men. It's up to us to keep our sexuality alive.

6

Timing Is Everything

....

I'M A CLOCK WATCHER. Ask anyone who knows me, I always seem to know what time it is. When I wake up in the morning, I guess the time, look at the clock, and voilà, I'm usually right. I keep wondering how this is possible. I suspect it's because, like all of us, I live my life by the clock. And as couples eager to conceive know only too well, fertility clock-watching is no exception.

Timing is the operative word for any woman who wants children. "Am I too old, did I waste too much time?" "Why is it taking so long to get pregnant?" "When is the right time to have sex?" are questions frequently asked in my practice. Needless to say, I spend a lot of time educating women.

CREATING SPACE, RELEASING FEAR

We want to make our womb, the sacred jade palace, receptive, and to do that we need to figure out what gets in the way of knowing when to rest and nourish and when to put our sexy on and get the fire started. More often than not, fear plays a role in our confusion. We must make space for all that we feel—and many women embarking on a fertility journey feel all the feelings from excitement to fear and back again, from joyful connection with a partner to anger, hurt, and despair. Some get stressed that their biological clock is ticking and then worry that the stress is compromising their fertility. They take the odds of conceiving naturally as gospel, listening to their doctors list statistics that dampen any hope they might have had: 20 to 25 percent chance (per month) for healthy women in their twenties; less than 10 percent by age thirty-five, and a scant 5 percent by age forty.

They're convinced they must think only positive baby-making thoughts or they'll fail to conceive, and yet they're obsessed with the what-ifs and the if-onlys. Such is the battle raging in their minds. The best way to calm the storm within is to stay present, and the best way to stay present is to understand what's really happening in your body and find ways to be in a relationship with it instead of at odds with it.

Let's begin with a quick review of the cycles of fertility according to both Western and Eastern medicine.

How It All Works

It all starts with menstruation. In Western medicine, twenty-six to thirty-two days is considered an average menstrual cycle, and not much emphasis is placed on when it begins, as long as it's regular. Taoists and Ayurvedic practitioners believe that to conceive women should bleed on the new moon, because that is the most yin and has empty energy, and they should ovulate on the full moon because that has the most yang, or full energy. Don't worry if that isn't how your cycle falls; you can still approach it the same way.

On the first day of your cycle, if you haven't conceived, falling levels of estrogen and progesterone will signal the endometrial lining to shed, and you will begin to bleed.

On days two to four, even as you continue to bleed, the endometrial lining begins to remodel and rebuild. This is the time to move inward, to rest, nourish yourself, be in nature, and commune with your female friends—and to mourn if you feel the sadness of not conceiving, forgiving your body, breathing love and spaciousness into your uterus, and committing to letting go as you shed what needs to be shed. By its very nature, a new cycle, which begins with the onset of your period, means a time to begin again. It is not the time, however, to have sex, because according to Chinese medicine, blood is flowing out, and you don't want push it back up in the act of intercourse. Instead, love and appreciate the magnificent gift of bleeding. Ayurveda agrees—this is the time of *apana vayu*, or "downward-moving energy." Instead, think of your menses as a natural cleanse, Ayurvedic practitioners say. Every twenty-six to thirty-two days, your body gathers all the detritus and toxins (called *ama* in Ayurveda) that have built up during the month and moves it out, along with menstrual blood.

THE FOLLICULAR PHASE: During this time and up until just before ovulation, an egg begins to mature within the ovaries. In this phase, estrogen reaches its peak and sets about preparing the body to conceive. Chinese medicine calls this the "yin phase" and in Ayurveda it's kapha time—the body is getting juicier and more receptive; it's building up strength and preparing to receive. Not only is the cervical fluid abundant, the uterine lining is also growing, creating a nice, receptive, nurturing home for a possible embryo. You may feel your emotions flow more freely now because yin and kapha both connect deeply to memories and emotions.

Now is the time to make love, make love, and make love. Reignite that spark that brought you two together in the first place. You can grab your ovulation predictor kit—the pee stick—and find out if you're ovulating now. Don't put too much stock in the pee stick, however; it doesn't always work. Personally, I never could make one work, but I knew my cycles were regular. I knew when I was ovulating because I paid attention to my cervical mucus, which becomes fertile as estrogen peaks—about two days before ovulation. You can tell because it resembles raw egg whites; sperm love it because fertile mucus changes the pH of the vagina, making it less acidic and more hospitable.

OVULATION: Once you begin ovulating, your body gives off all kinds of signals that it's ready to make things happen. The cervix shifts from its low position to a higher one in the body, which conveniently provides a bit more room for intercourse. You may be wetter vaginally and feel that sex is deeper. And, not coincidentally, during this time your sex drive increases. You feel hot, sexy, and alive!

THE LUTEAL PHASE: Approximately fourteen days between ovulation and beginning of menstruation, this phase is generally the most reliable. This is when progesterone is produced, causing the uterine lining—the endometrium—to secrete nutrients for conception. It then switches off hormones that would ripen more eggs and triggers small blood vessels to produce more blood flow to your endometrium. Chinese medicine describes this phase as being yang in nature—warming and active; in Ayurveda it's the pitta phase—fiery and transformative.

If you've been taking your basal body temperature, expect it to rise slightly (usually between four-tenths of a degree and one degree higher than the follicular phase temperature). Now is when implantation of an embryo can occur—six to ten days after ovulation—which could mean success.

Many of my female patients say they are afraid of having sex or an orgasm during the luteal phase because they think that it might dislodge an implanted embryo. If the embryo's healthy and you're healthy, you needn't worry—it's pretty unlikely that having sex or an orgasm would cause the little one to escape its comfy room in the womb. Of course, if you have any doubts, check with your doctor first. A 2016 study suggests that seminal fluid positively affects the female reproductive tract and can even bolster immune response.[1]

So if your cycle marches along as nature intends, you can predict with some degree of accuracy when you will ovulate. However, what happens when your cycle has a mind of its own? Andy Huang, MD, who specializes in reproductive endocrinology and infertility (REI) at Reproductive Partners Medical Group in Los Angeles, is one of those rare doctors who actually educates his patients about their cycles. He reminds his patients that nature is unpredictable and women needn't worry unless their menstrual cycles are never regular. If that's the case, we need to figure out what's going on. Conditions such as polycystic ovarian syndrome (PCOS) can interfere with ovulation. But sometimes there's no rhyme or reason for irregular cycles. Acupuncture, herbs, and nutritional supplements often help regulate a cycle that is out of whack.

What happens if your ovulation window isn't open like it usually is? Here's a scenario: You've counted the days until ovulation and you're sure it's time. You've taken care of everything, planned an intimate evening with your beloved, however, the pee stick doesn't indicate you are ovulating. What could be happening? If you normally ovulate on a regular schedule, it could be a faulty pee stick. But truly, lots of things can conspire to alter ovulation, including stress, travel, a change in medication, hormonal fluctuations, and illness. Be gentle with yourself; this could simply be a one-time occurrence and nothing to worry about.

SO, WHAT ABOUT SEX?

I can't tell you how often I've been asked if there's a magic number of times to have sex when a woman's ovulating. Even more astounding, I often have to gently remind some of my patients that they really do need to have sex if they want to have a baby. But how much sex and when, and how do you talk about it so it doesn't feel like an obligation or your partner doesn't resent you? It's such a complicated issue because the urgency to conceive puts added pressure on both partners to get it on—even as it brings up myriad questions on when to and how to.

How *do* you let your partner know "it's time," without making the whole thing feel like an obligation, an inconvenience, or a chore? That's the million-dollar question most women want answered. Just like everything else, you have to talk about these things together because you're in this together, remember? Get to know your partner. Some men want to know all the physiological details of a woman's cycle—it makes them feel like they're participating in the journey. But for the majority of men who come to my office, seeing a positive ovulation test kit can be an anxiety-producing turnoff.

First order of business is to educate your partner about your cycle—preferably before you're in the middle of ovulating. Explain what fertile cervical mucus feels like and let him know how many days after your cycle you normally ovulate so he can calculate when the right time is himself, if he wants to. Of course, don't forget to ask him how he would like to know when you're in your fertile window. I decided to ask some of my male patients what works for them, and here are some of their answers:

> **I work a lot so I like to be prepared.** I told my wife I want to know when she gets a positive pee stick reading, so she sends me a happy face emoji while I'm work. It's a lighthearted gesture that helps me get in the mood for later that evening.

I keep a calendar of my wife's cycles—and I love doing it. I'm the one who says, "Honey, isn't it your ovulation time?" She's a busy executive and loves that I'm the one who keeps track of this.

I don't want to know the exact day my partner is ovulating—too clinical—but I can tell because she's wetter during that time.

I hate to feel pressure to perform and my partner knows that. So we decided that from day eight of her cycle onward we would have sex every other day. And we agreed to try to have fun with it. The good news is that we both like to have sex. Sure, sometimes we're tired and maybe not in the mood, but we just laugh.

Now that you're both well-versed on the whole fertile-window scheduling thing, the next question is how often should you make love during that window? That depends. And guys, this is where you come in. It depends on a number of factors, not the least of which is the quality of your sperm. Before explaining, I must point out that many men who have been told that their sperm count is too low are still able to impregnate their partners. But generally speaking, fertility experts focus on three parameters (out of many) for assessing the odds of success:

1. **Sperm count:** How many sperm are in each milliliter of semen? The range for what's considered normal is quite broad—anywhere from 40 to 300 million sperm per milliliter of semen. According to World Health Organization (WHO) guidelines, at least 20 million parts per milliliter are necessary for conception to occur, while studies show that men with at least 40 to 50 million/ml have the best chances. Those whose count is down to 15 million/ml are considered subfertile.

2. **Sperm motility:** Quantity isn't everything. Men also need to have sperm that are good swimmers—at least 32 percent of them, according to WHO guidelines. These are the powerful swimmers that can make the long journey toward an egg. One of my patients came into my office looking dejected. His doctor ran a sperm test on him and found that most of his sperm were swimming slowly. As it turned out, this man's daily marijuana habit was affecting his sperms' motility.

Luckily, after he stopped smoking for three months, his sperm began to move a little faster.

3. **Sperm morphology:** It's not enough that you've got enough sperm and they can swim. Size and shape matter, too. Using a strict semen analysis (called "Kruger strict criteria"), specialized labs can determine whether your sperm morphology puts you at risk of infertility. Unlike the WHO guidelines that are based on population studies, Kruger strict criteria are based on what the sperm actually look like. The criteria have found that in a given sample of ejaculate, at least 4 percent should be normal—the heads should be oval and the sperm should be sporting just one tail, not two. Sounds weird, I know, but men do produce some odd-looking sperm. Luckily, only between 4 and 14 percent need to be good-looking enough to penetrate an egg.

Many IVF centers now use what's called an "intracytoplasmic sperm injection," or ICSI, which allows technicians to choose sperm to inject into an egg. There's good news for men who have compromised sperm numbers, lazy swimmers, or oddly shaped sperm, however: according to recent studies, even men who have 0 percent normal morphology can still impregnate their partners naturally.[2] So morphology alone cannot be used to predict fertilization, pregnancy, or live birth potential. Reproductive urologist Paul Turek, an expert in men's reproductive and sexual health, agrees that size and shape of sperm isn't everything. He says that "simply eyeballing the sperm as good- or bad-looking doesn't really reflect what's going on inside (i.e., genetic payload). It's really judging the book by its cover."[3]

Another bit of good news, guys, is that semen and the sperm it contains can change. Your body produces sperm approximately every seventy days. While it's true that illness, certain medications, prior surgeries, genetics, hormones, and such lifestyle choices as smoking, excessive alcohol consumption, overexercising, and chronic stress can have a negative effect on sperm, consciously changing what you can change can often have a positive influence.

Of course, it doesn't hurt for you to get your sperm tested if you and your partner haven't been able to conceive after six months to a year or more of trying. If your sperm isn't good, ask your doctor about DNA fragmentation testing, which measures the degree of damage to the sperm. Male infertility specialist Dr. Philip Werthman says, "In my vast experience using sperm DNA fragmentation testing, I have found it to be one of the most reliable predictors of fertility, and we use this test frequently."[4]

So now that we've covered sperm parameters, let's get back to having sex. Most physicians recommend baby-making sex about every other day during the fertile six-day window. Paul Magarelli, MD, a reproductive endocrinologist and infertility specialist from HQA Fertility Centers in Colorado Springs, Colorado, believes that having intercourse twice a week, separated by two days, should cover fertility timing 100 percent. Why? "Because sperm can live up to four to five days in the female genital tract and eggs live up to forty-eight hours after ovulation," he says. "So, it's very hard to miss with this timing."[5] Another reproductive endocrinology and infertility expert, Catherine DeUgarte, MD, agrees. "Intercourse should ideally occur two to three times around ovulation," she says. "The highest probability of conception occurs one day before or on the day of ovulation."

Ejaculating every two to three days keeps sperm healthy. Waiting too long increases the chances of having more dead, immotile, or morphologically abnormal sperm. When I asked Dr. Werthman what his recommendations were for men whose sperm parameters are low, he replied, "If a man has high levels of DNA fragmentation, then ejaculating more frequently can be beneficial. But if he has a very low sperm count, it may be detrimental."

Now that you've checked everything out, the next thing is to actually have sex. Make love! You think I'm kidding, but honestly, the complaint I hear so often is that "we rarely make love anymore. I'm so tired from working and then stressing over all of this fertility stuff that the last thing that interests me is having sex. We never had sex during the week, but now that having a baby is a priority, I guess we have to."

We have to. Those three words just removed any connection between baby-making sex and intimacy. The *we have to* complaint has relegated sex to a chore, a have-to, a means to an end. Of course, I get it that everyone's sexual appetite is different, but that's not the point. The point is that you've entered into this covenant because you want to share your love with another little being; you want that little being to be the outcome of a loving connection. To do that, you need to rekindle that connection. Remember when having sex was something both you and your partner couldn't get enough of? All those feel-good hormones—who doesn't want that? Get back to that. Sex can be fun, even if it's a quickie or a pick-me-up when you're tired.

It may sound like a cliché, but just setting aside time to connect and be together, with no goal in mind, helps. I know it's not quite like the "I can't get enough of you" sex you had when you were first together, but it can at least get the party started. Remember, there are times when the sex is hot and heavy and other times when it is a deep, quiet, and loving connection. It's all okay. Of course, if you're not really feeling it and think you've lost your mojo, give chapter 7 a read for ideas on how to improve your sex drive.

TIMING SEX USING WESTERN REPRODUCTIVE MEDICINE

Where the timing of sexual intercourse gets tricky—and confusing—is during in vitro fertilization (IVF) and other forms of reproductive assisted medicine. I've heard it all—from no sex (and by "sex," most doctors mean penetration) for twelve full weeks after implantation of an embryo (which seems extreme) to sex up till the first ultrasound. I remember being with one of my patients to whom I had just given pre-IVF transfer acupuncture. A nurse came in, had her sign some forms, and then gave her a handout on how to care for herself during the ten days post-transfer. The instructions explicitly said "no intercourse." "What does that even mean," she asked me? She had so many questions and no one to answer them. "Can I have oral sex, anal sex? What if I have an orgasm, is that okay? Can I masturbate?" I needed to clear up the confusion myself, so I arranged to talk with various specialists in reproductive endocrinology and infertility. I started with Richard Marrs, MD, the leading REI at California Fertility Partners in Los Angeles, who began by talking about sex *before* egg-retrieval time.

I asked Dr. Marrs whether someone doing an IVF could have intercourse and whether she could have ejaculate in her vagina. "Sperm in the system is not a problem," he said. "They can have intercourse anytime—up until around the egg recovery, when the ovaries become quite enlarged. The reason for this is because the ovaries are heavy and have multiple follicles on them; if the woman has active sex with her partner, the ovaries can sometimes twist." He went on to tell me, "Women can have more discomfort with intercourse two to three days before an egg recovery and four to five days after the egg collection, when the ovaries are still enlarged and more tender. So we tell couples to avoid intercourse two to three days before and up to a week after."

That timing works well because if the couple is using the partner's sperm, he will need to avoid ejaculating two days before retrieval and make sure he "cleans the pipes" (ejaculates) not more than three days (seventy-two hours) before making his deposit. Men should not go more than five to seven days without ejaculation because there can be a high percentage of dead sperm. Of course, there are exceptions. Men with low sperm counts may need only two days of abstinence before giving samples to produce better-quality sperm.

What I will say is beware of the internet and don't believe everything you Google. For example, I recently saw a message from a viewer of a sex and IVF video. The viewer's question was "Can you have sex during fertility treatment?" The answer stunned me: "Here is the bad news, sex really isn't a good idea during treatment. . . . The no-sex rule starts the moment you decide to start treatment." That's just wrong. Many other sites reported that women don't even want to have sex during their IVF journey. That's also wrong. For some women, sex doesn't appeal, but others crave sex.

One of my patients, Judy, looked at me on day five of her fertility shots and said, "I have so much cervical fluid, I just want to have sex all day long, but can I? If not, is masturbation okay?" I must say, I appreciated her candor.

When I spoke to Carolyn Alexander, MD, an REI specialist at the Southern California Reproductive Center, she helped clarify all of this. She said that after egg retrieval, where a 16-gauge needle pokes through the vaginal wall to the follicle to collect the egg, there is a hole that will close in twenty-four hours. Therefore, no intercourse during that time because of the risk of infection from the ejaculate. Ovarian torsion (twisting) can also occur during intercourse, even if the man doesn't ejaculate in the cavity before the egg retrieval, and there is a risk of hemorrhage from each follicle which can be filled with blood. When women have a frozen embryo transfer (FET), Dr. Alexander allows orgasm but no penetration because the uterus can contract with deep penetration, she says. Although other REIs don't have such stringent guidelines—and there's currently not enough supportive research—Dr. Alexander says she doesn't want ejaculate in the uterine cavity after a frozen embryo transfer or close to the time of the transfer either. She says that ejaculate can carry bacteria (ureaplasma, mycoplasma) or even bacteria from the intestine (enterococcus), which shouldn't mingle with vaginal microbiota (i.e., microscopic organisms).

Part of the confusion stems from the fact that there are several different Western medicine fertility protocols for women and men. These protocols depend on many factors, including age, hormone status, anatomy, physiology, and whether a woman is using donor eggs, donor sperm, and/ or a surrogate. I can't cover all these factors here, but I can give a quick rundown on the sex specifics or at least what we know of them. There isn't a lot of research in this area, although new studies are happening all the time, so most of what follows is a compilation of knowledge from many clinics around the nation and abroad. Every stimulation protocol is different, but they do have some common features.

Downregulation (IVF only)

In this protocol, a woman is put on an oral contraceptive pill (OCP) or gonadotropin-releasing hormone agonist (GnRH agonist) such as Lupron so that her ovaries will turn off temporarily. Not all protocols use these drugs.

RECOMMENDATIONS: Intercourse, oral sex, anal sex, and clitoral stimulation all get a green light for women. Some doctors advocate using condoms because Lupron is considered teratogenic, which means it can disturb the development of an embryo. Men: all good up until the few days before you're ready to give your sample.

CAVEATS: Some women may not feel like having sex, especially those who get hit with any side effects of Lupron—hot flashes, night sweats, headache, insomnia, and gastrointestinal distress. But there is always loving touch and holding each other.

Injectable Stimulation Drugs

These are used for both intrauterine inseminations (IUI) and in vitro fertilization (IVF). Dosage is generally lower for an IUI. Gonadotropins like Follistim, Gonal-F, Menopur, Bravelle, and others stimulate the ovaries to make follicles that contain eggs.

SIDE EFFECTS: usually mild for most women, including headache, nausea, fatigue, bloating, and enlarged ovaries

RECOMMENDATIONS FOR IVF: Intercourse, oral sex, clitoral stimulation, and orgasm—all with caveats. Intercourse, some say, should end on day four of shots; others say it's fine up until two to three days before retrieval; and still others say no intercourse at all while injecting. All experts say intercourse is not advised if the ovaries are very enlarged because of the risk of ovarian torsion. Most doctors agree that you should refrain from oral sex twenty-four hours before retrieval, but they admit that no research exists to support this caution. Clitoral stimulation and orgasm is fine until retrieval.

RECOMMENDATIONS FOR IUI: Intercourse, oral sex, anal sex, clitoral stimulation, and orgasm are all fine, but check with your doctor to make sure your ovaries are not enlarged, as penetration can increase the risk of ovarian torsion. If you are using your partner's sperm, he should not go more than five days without ejaculating; however, he should refrain two to three days before giving his sample.

Oral Stimulation Drugs

These drugs—the most common of which is Clomid—are used to stimulate more follicles in women who either don't ovulate or who have other fertility challenges. They are sometimes given along with injectables for IVF.

SIDE EFFECTS: Mood swings, vaginal dryness, hot flashes, abdominal discomfort, visual disturbances, ovarian cyst formation, nausea, thinning of the endometrial lining, and reduced production of cervical mucus. Because Clomid is an antiestrogen drug, many women report greater side effects with it than with injectables.

RECOMMENDATIONS: No limits on sex. However, since vaginal dryness can be a side effect, women may want to use a lubricant. Make sure to choose a lube that is indicated for fertility (see chapter 14). As with injectables, if you are using your partner's sperm he should not go more than five days without ejaculating, but refrain two to three days before giving his sample.

Egg Retrieval

Recommendations vary from clinic to clinic, but when there are multiple eggs taken out, some practitioners err on the side of caution and say no vaginal intercourse for seven to ten days, up to two weeks, after retrieval. Orgasms might be fine, although they may not be what you want to do right now. Of course, always check with your doctor if you're experiencing any discomfort, bleeding, or complications, such as ovarian hyperstimulation, which can be serious. Eric Surrey, MD, a board-certified REI at the Colorado Center for Reproductive Medicine, says, "If embryos are frozen, no intercourse for two weeks after retrieval until first menses to avoid infection as well as concern for ovarian torsion or bleeding."

Egg Donors

No unprotected sex one week before and one week after egg retrieval, Dr. Marrs cautions, to guard against any leftover egg in the system that could get picked up by a fallopian tube and cause the donor to become pregnant.

Intrauterine Insemination (IUI)

Recommendations apply whether a couple is using injectable drugs, oral drugs, or no drugs at all.

RECOMMENDATIONS: Most doctors encourage intercourse, especially the evening of the IUI because studies show that the semen in the female reproductive tract enhances the uterine lining, making it more receptive to the embryo attaching itself there.

Post-Implantation after in Vitro Fertilization (IVF) or Frozen Embryo Transfer (FET)

Guidelines are all over the place, so check with your doctor.

RECOMMENDATIONS: Generally speaking, doctors will say you should be on "pelvic rest" anywhere from five days to two weeks after a transfer. Pelvic rest is a polite way of saying no intercourse, no hanky-panky of any kind. It used to be that doctors wanted their patients to not only be on pelvic rest, but on bed rest, too. But according to guidelines from the American Society of Reproductive Medicine, bed rest makes no difference in pregnancy outcomes, so it's not necessary. Pelvic rest seems a bit extreme to me, so I decided to ask a few reproductive specialists to weigh in.

First up, Dr. Surrey agreed that for IVF, you should "avoid intercourse or orgasm beginning with the embryo transfer and extending until the first normal pregnancy ultrasound exam, about six weeks." When I asked him if manual or oral stimulation would be okay, he said, "Orgasm would be a theoretic concern because of the potential of uterine contractions, although there is no data to support that."

Is it really true that an orgasm can cause strong enough uterine contractions to dislodge an embryo? When I asked Dr. Marrs about clitoral and vaginal orgasms in and around embryo implantation (either naturally occurring or using IVF and FET), he said, "The answer is no one really knows. I tell couples, if they want to be conservative, orgasms a week after transfer are okay." He went on to say what I had hoped he would: "To be totally honest with you, if that was critical, none of us would be here, because in natural conception you have orgasm; an embryo implants, then you have an orgasm again. Once implantation has taken place, uterine contractions are not going to spit out an embryo that is half a millimeter in size. Highly unlikely."

Positive Pregnancy Test

The following is advice for couples undergoing IVF or FET, as well as those who got pregnant the natural way.

RECOMMENDATIONS FOR IVF AND FET: Now that you've been successful, some clinics will recommend that you avoid intercourse until you hear the baby's heartbeat. Others say that having sex is fine two weeks after implantation. Because there's a higher risk in assisted reproduction of ectopic pregnancy—where the egg is implanted outside of the uterus, most often in a fallopian tube—Dr. DeUgarte says she usually "waits for the first ultrasound to make sure the pregnancy is not ectopic." If the ovaries are still enlarged during a new cycle, no intercourse is recommended.

All Couples (Natural and Assisted)

Avoid intercourse if there is bleeding or any other worrisome condition. And to be doubly sure, ask your clinic about their recommendations. Again, once an embryo has implanted, there's no reason to believe that having intercourse or an orgasm (causing uterine contractions) would dislodge an embryo. However, if you have a history of miscarriage or signs that the uterine lining isn't stable, or if you're nervous about anything, don't have intercourse that first trimester.

So what's a couple to make of all this? Certainly those who are going the medically assisted route have more to negotiate regarding sex. When I asked Jani White, an acupuncturist in the UK and the author of *The Fertile Fizz*, about her opinion on sex during IVF, she said, "Sex for women doing IVF isn't always high on their list of things they feel like doing—they're probably constipated, bloated, nervous, and not feeling particularly desirable." So instead, Jani encourages her couples to practice what she calls "cherishment." I love that idea. Cherish. Your. Partner. What a wonderful concept. "Baby hormones need to get up to speed by stroking, hand-holding, making eye contact, and showering together," she says, all of which "will increase [a woman's] oxytocin, and that should help her conceive. Understand that the chemistry of attraction is the chemistry of conception."

SEXUAL SECRET
An Ancient Chinese Method for Choosing the Sex of Your Baby

Want to have a little fun? The Chinese sages say you can predict the sex of your baby even before conception by using Chinese astrology. You take your date of birth, the year you'd like to conceive, and the gender you'd like your baby to be, and plug all of that into an online Chinese astrological calendar. You'll want to find a site that converts your information from the Gregorian calendar to the Chinese luna-solar calendar. My patient Lily swears it works! When she and her husband were trying for their second, they wanted to have a girl because they already had a boy. And sure enough, by using this method they had a girl.

Of course, it's just for fun. If we concern ourselves with our baby's sex we'll miss the beautiful nature of the unknown. Although I wonder how it would work with IVF . . .

7

Fine-Tuning the Engine

....

The best way to get things done is simply to begin.

—CHARLENE ADAMS

THE HEALTHIER YOU ARE—mentally, emotionally, and physically—the better your odds of having (or even wanting to have) great sex, and the more likely you'll conceive. Luckily, taking a serious look at your lifestyle and then making some healthy changes can help you fire up your sex drive and rekindle a more loving connection. We already know how a distorted body image and the usual destructive habits (smoking, alcohol, drugs) can squash desire. So now let's see how more conscious habits can nourish life, support a loving relationship, and bring things back into balance. In other words, let's get practical. The best way I know to approach this subject is through the lens of the five elements of traditional Chinese medicine (TCM) and Taoist philosophy: earth, metal, wood, water, and fire.

Taoists believe that *yang sheng*, which means "nourishing life," increases health and longevity. To do that, the Tao asks us to live in harmony with nature and balance our sleep, diet, exercise, and spiritual practices.

THE EARTH ELEMENT: ATTENDING TO YOUR CENTER

The earth is at the center of the five elements and constitutes the core of our being. A strong center means a healthy digestion. A healthy digestive tract can more easily extract nutrients from the foods you eat, which are necessary for nutrition and to potentially increase the health of the follicles in your ovaries (or the number and motility of sperm in your testicles). A balanced earth element means living in harmony with the planet, feeling centered in your body, and caring and nurturing yourself. In addition, you are present in the moment, with ample energy, because you are no longer beset by worries and fears. They don't call women ready to conceive Earth Mothers for nothing!

Being Present in the Body

There is nothing sexier than a woman or man who is comfortable in their body. What does it mean to love yourself *exactly as you are?* Jessica Durivage, a yoga instructor and a self-described "wildly authentic truth-weaver," is the founder of Every Woman's Voice, an intimate online learning center. She told me that her practice of yoga nidra (a powerful meditation technique that promotes deep rest and relaxation, described in chapter 12), ecstatic dance, and caring for and healing her womb (the second chakra) has made for the best sex. "Nothing has changed with my partner," she says, "but I have changed." So often a preoccupation with our looks, our bellies, the size of our penis, or the shape of our vulvas gets in the way of intimacy and good sex. Earth energy calls for you to meet yourself with love—and without judgment—and this includes the body that your soul inhabits.

Those with earth imbalance often need and seek the approval of others. They tend to feel ungrounded and a bit alienated from their physical bodies. Women whose bodies are going through a medically assisted fertility journey find it especially hard to celebrate their physicality or believe that they're desirable. It does help to remember these changes are temporary, and they are happening in service to your ultimate goal.

Gabrielle Roth, an American dancer and creator of the 5Rhythms approach to movement, said it best: "Your body is the ground metaphor of your life, the expression of your existence. . . . So many of us are not in our bodies, really at home and vibrantly present there. Nor are we in touch with the basic rhythms that constitute our bodily life. We live outside our-selves . . . in our heads, our memories, our longings . . . absentee landlords of our own estate. . . . My way back into life was ecstatic dance. I re-entered my body by learning to move myself, to dance my own dance from the inside out, not the outside in."[1]

Earth-Balancing Diet: Western Approach

So, what is the best food strategy for maximizing conception and feeling your best sexy self? Easiest thing to remember: eat fresh, preferably organic and locally grown foods as much as possible. Cut out refined, processed foods, sugar, and hydrogenated fats—anything that produces an inflammatory response in the body. Many holistic nutritionists and fertility specialists recommend giving up wheat products for this very reason. In their book *Feed Your Fertility*, my colleagues Emily Bartlett and Laura Erlich say that "improperly prepared grains are likely to contribute to inflammation—exacerbating painful periods, hormone imbalance and other symptoms of inflammation and pain." They go on to say that if you do eat grains, you should choose "beans and nuts that have first been soaked, sprouted, or soured."[2] David Perlmutter, an integrative neurologist and the author of *Grain Brain*, believes we should eliminate *all* grains and instead focus on healthy fats—extra-virgin olive oil, coconut oil, and grass-fed butter; protein-rich food, including wild fish, grass-fed meat, and hormone-free chicken and tofu; and plenty of vegetables and a modest amount of low sugar, stone-bearing fruits.

With these guidelines in mind, eat foods that feel good and shy away from anything that compromises your digestion. For example, if after eating tofu you feel gassy and bloated, soy products may not be a good option for you—or you may want to try fermented soy products instead, such as natto, tempeh, or miso. To increase fertility, some nutritionists insist that you get enough omega-3 fatty acids. If you're not a vegetarian, cold-water oily fish or supplements are your best bet; vegetarians should eat more walnuts and flaxseed or look for microalgae supplements. If you're eating fish, make sure that is sustainable and not high in mercury or other toxins.

Earth-Balancing Diet: Eastern Approach

In Chinese medicine, we prescribe dietary changes by first identifying the patient's constitution and imbalances and then recommending foods accordingly. For example, if a patient craves sweets, is often bloated and tired, has loose stools, is plagued with allergies, and has a thick tongue coating, we diagnose this person as a Spleen qi and dampness type. The specific dietary recommendations would include avoiding dairy, sweets, and raw foods. Generally, with a condition like this, TCM practitioners say avoid eating cold and raw foods like iced drinks, salads, and sandwiches, which can be harmful to Spleen energy, especially during your menstrual cycle. They believe that a "cold womb" is one of the reasons for infertility, and it can often be the result of eating primarily cold, raw foods.

In her book *Cooking for Fertility*, nutritional consultant Kathryn Simmons Flynn breaks down the different Chinese pattern imbalances and gives specific recipe recommendations for each. When I asked her what types of foods and spices she recommends to increase fertility and revitalize sexual desire, she had a whole list that included ginger, cinnamon, salmon (or other cold-water omega-rich seafood), chlorophyll, cloves, fenugreek seeds, fennel seeds, anise seeds, black peppercorn, walnuts, black beans, and dark chocolate.

Ayurveda, the ancient Indian practice of medicine, also looks at the whole person when assessing fertility. Niika Quistgard, an Ayurvedic practitioner and wellness educator, says she likes to see where the biggest imbalances are, and she prefers to focus on what's happening right now. If you were to see her she'd evaluate your nervous system, digestive system, mental-emotional state, stress level, and food intake. She would want to know *when* you eat, as well as *what* you eat—is it cooked or is it raw?—and how strong your digestion is. In India, where she worked at a women's clinic, women and men go through a cleanse called *pancha karma* to prepare for conception. That process typically lasts between three and six months, although in the States there are shorter, less intense options.

One More Reason to Nurture Your Belly

Whether you adhere to a Western or an Eastern approach to a healthy diet, the bottom line is that you must eat foods that promote healthy gut function and a healthy microbiome in your mouth, skin, gut, and in the reproductive organs of both sexes (including the vagina, penis, and the man's urogenital tract). A healthy microbiome benefits gut health and the immune system and keeps your hormone levels balanced. Each one of us has a unique microbiome that contains ten times more microbes than it does regular cells. Notably, if you're pregnant, the same microorganisms present in your mouth are also found in your placenta. The microbes in your vagina are passed along to your baby through the birth canal, so keeping that microbiome healthy is vital. Even if you give birth by C-section, you can still "seed the microbiome of the baby with [your] normal vaginal flora," according to Barbara Harper, RN, a midwife and the founder of Waterbirth International. You can do this by swabbing your vagina with your hand and putting your hand in your newborn's mouth and rubbing his or her skin.

Just like every other part of your body, your vaginal microbiome benefits from eating fresh, organic food and adding small amounts of fermented foods. As well, you should stay away from sugar and other refined foods, manage your stress and worry, take a probiotic supplement, and be careful about what products you put into your vagina. Choose organic, natural cotton tampons and pads during menses and avoid lubricants that contain glycerin or synthetic fragrances (chapter 14 goes into more detail about lubricants). And if you douche, please stop, as this can kill off beneficial vaginal flora.

Prebiotic foods are also important to add to your diet. These nondigestible fiber compounds feed the beneficial microorganisms in the intestines. They include chicory root (a great coffee substitute), dandelion greens, asparagus, alliums (garlic, onions, leeks, and chives), jicama, and Jerusalem artichokes. Registered dietitian Robyn Goldberg says contrary to popular opinion, it's fine to lightly cook prebiotics instead of always consuming them raw. Adding some digestive enzymes to your supplement regimen can also be beneficial.

Earth Element Emotions: Don't Worry, Be Happy

Chinese medicine says that overthinking and overworrying damage Spleen and Stomach energies, which are governed by the earth element; therefore, avoid emotional extremes. When you worry about the timing of intercourse, about successful outcomes, about your future, you may actually be making things worse. In the same way that we're careful about what we feed our body, we must be careful about how we feed our mind. Gentle yoga practice, conscious breathing, laughter, journaling, and simply being together without an agenda can all contribute to a healthy mind and therefore a healthy womb.

SEXY FOODS

Asparagus

Psychologist Linda De Villers, who specializes in human sexuality and is the author of *Simply Sexy Food: 101 Tasty Aphrodisiac Recipes and Sensual Tips to Stir Your Libido and Feed Your Love*, says, "In French, the word *asperge* is slang for penis. Nineteenth-century French bridegrooms were mandated to eat several courses of asparagus on the wedding eve to assure the groom of sexual stamina (and in the Renaissance, it was recommended for 'timid' newlyweds)."[3]

Chocolate

Chocolate contains all kind of sexy: theobromine, a nervous system stimulant similar to caffeine that gets your energy up; small quantities of phenylethylamine (PEA), the same chemical that gets released in the brain when you fall in love; and anandamide, an endocannabinoid, your brain's own bliss hormone. In fact, anandamide, found in dark chocolate and raw chocolate, shares the same receptors that cannabis binds to. Opt for raw or dark chocolate and feel free to add herbs that increase libido such as maca, horny goat weed, yohimbe, damiana, and ashwagandha.

Garlic

In Ayurvedic medicine, garlic is considered stimulating and can increase sexual desire—taboo if you're celibate, but for the rest of us, pretty great news. Studies show that garlic contains substances that relax the blood vessels that increase blood flow to the genitals—important for erections, both clitoral and penile. So, put a trip to an Italian restaurant on the calendar and don't worry about garlic breath!

Goji Berries

Considered an herb in Chinese medicine, these little red "happy" berries are high in antioxidants and are known to boost energy as well as sperm count, and help prevent premature ovarian failure.

Pineapple

If you are doing an IVF, ask someone to bring you a pineapple right after your embryo transfer. Why? Because pineapple contains the anti-inflammatory enzyme bromelain—mostly in its stem—so eating it may help with embryo implantation. But how does pineapple translate to sexy? Feeding each other juicy pineapple sections can be a whole lot of messy fun and could maybe lead to even more fun—under the sheets!

Pumpkin Seeds

High in zinc, pumpkin seeds may increase testosterone and semen levels. Add them to your goji berries for a good trail mix. For women, try seed cycling by ingesting one tablespoon of pumpkin seeds and one tablespoon of flaxseeds from the end of the period until ovulation to help balance estrogen.

Shellfish

Oysters contain more zinc per serving than any other food, and zinc is great for men's sexual function. D-aspartic acid, a component of bivalve mollusks (oysters, clams, mussels, and scallops), is an amino acid that has been shown to increase the level of sex hormones in lab rats and may boost testosterone as well; it may also be good for women as zinc is also good for developing follicles.[4]

THE METAL ELEMENT: AWAKENING OUR ANIMAL NATURE

A rock, a stone, and a crystal all carry energies absorbed from many years on this planet, the metal in them shaped by life itself in its ever-changing currents. Similarly, our lives are given to us by the physical energies of our parents and shaped by our current circumstances. We inherit mitochondria (the energy cells in our body) from our mothers and, in accordance with Chinese medicine, we also inherit the animal spirit of the metal energy, called *po*. Po permeates our physical being and awakens our body. One aspect of this energy manifests as our animal nature—wild, untamed, and primal—represented in that frantic time in a relationship when we just want to tear each other's clothes off. It is this energy that makes the cells grow into an embryo.

Unfortunately, if you are doing assisted reproductive medicine such as IVF, you may need a little help creating the metal energy your cells need to divide and grow. Some experts suggest taking a CoEnzyme Q_{10} supplement—a powerful antioxidant that may increase fertility in both women and men. Ample CoQ_{10} in the follicular fluid, some studies have suggested, results in higher pregnancy rates.[5] Because of its antioxidant properties and its ability to help mitochondrial function, CoQ_{10} also may play a positive role in sperm health and motility.

Metal Element Emotions: Letting Go and De-Armoring

The metal element manifests in the lungs and the large intestine, both of which pertain to taking in and letting go. In all traditions, the breath is considered the pathway to optimal physical, emotional, and spiritual health. Focusing on the breath—particularly the exhalation—allows us to settle and come back to the present moment. We can use the breath in this way to surrender and de-armor ourselves. When we armor ourselves we put up a barrier to intimacy, exactly like putting on a coat of armor. De-armoring helps us let go of the need for protection because we feel secure in who we are. People who have been abused and hurt often armor different parts of themselves because of the pain they feel—they literally cut themselves off from experiencing pleasure.

According to Chinese medicine, grief is an emotion of the metal element and is stored in the lungs. Obviously, many couples trying to conceive experience grief, whether because of miscarriage or because of deep longing and disappointment each time pregnancy doesn't occur. When we refuse to acknowledge, investigate, and feel our emotions, they get lodged in the body and can surface as muscle tension and trauma, as well as other physical and emotional challenges. Therapy can certainly help, especially therapy that has a body-based component that allows you to move the sensations through and out of the body. (The exercises in chapter 8 are designed to move energy in this way.)

Metal Element: Toxins

Another manifestation of the metal element (and by extension, the lungs) in Chinese medicine is the skin. Our skin is the largest of our sensory organs. It is how we feel and communicate the full range of human emotions as well as register practical information like heat and cold and pain. It is also how we receive sensual and erotic pleasure. Caring for the skin is vital to health, therefore choose products that nurture the skin and stay away from toxic products that can damage it. Damaging the skin can deregulate the endocrine and nervous systems and wreak havoc on fertility and overall health. Remember, what you put *on* your body is just as important as what you put *in* it.

Toxins show up in the foods we eat, of course, which is why buying organic is so important. For example, dioxins, which are byproducts from industrial processes that build up in the fat cells of animals are particularly insidious and can show up in breast milk and in the placenta. If you eat animal products, choose only organic, free-range, pastured products. Avoid processed foods and anything that has been exposed to pesticides, and don't microwave your food.

Toxins are also present in many skin-care products and household cleaners. For a complete list of what to use and what to avoid, check out the Skin Deep database, from the Environmental Working Group (ewg. org/skindeep). It lists and rates products by how healthy they are for the body and the planet; just enter your favorite product in their database, and it will tell you whether it's safe and healthy to use. A couple of important considerations: if you can, either stop dyeing your hair or switch to a vegetable-based, nonperoxide hair dye. Switch from perfume, which is often laden with chemicals, to pure essential oils, which can calm or stimulate you naturally.

CIGARETTES: I can't believe we still need to talk about why cigarette smoking isn't a good idea when you're wanting to have a baby. And, seriously, my patients know it's not—even those who indulge. I remember one patient who tried to mask the stale smell that lingered on her clothes and in her hair with mints and rather strong perfume. I obviously had to say something. She protested that she worked out every day, ate really healthy foods, and even meditated. All great stuff, I told her, but here are the facts: according to the American Society of Reproductive Medicine (ASRM), cigarettes can increase erectile dysfunction, damage genetic material in eggs and sperm, and increase the chance of birth defects and ectopic pregnancy—and preterm labor occurs more often among female smokers.

CANNABIS: What about lighting up some weed? I know many couples who say it loosens them up and enhances desire. Studies are mixed and at the end of the day not very conclusive. Some research suggests that pot may negatively influence the size and shape of sperm and that hormones such as luteinizing hormone (LH) and testosterone could be also affected.[6] While cannabis doesn't appear to cause long-term fertility problems, it still makes sense to hold off, particularly since it lowers sperm counts by up to 55 percent, says reproductive urologist Paul Turek. And you may want to bracket your use of CBD oil, the nonpsychoactive ingredient in cannabis, until we know more about its effects on fertility and on the baby in utero.

THE WOOD ELEMENT: AWAKENING THE IMAGINATION

Out with the old, in with the new. The wood element is associated with springtime; it's all about new beginnings and outward expansion. Its energy manifests in the liver, which filters and moves toxins through and out of the body—the byproducts of the food we eat, our polluted environment, and the sometimes toxic emotions and relationships we experience. People with dominant wood energy are visionaries, connected to their dreams and imagination. When the wood element is compromised, emotions such as anger, frustration, blame, and shame build up and become stagnant, resulting in illness. Hormonal imbalance is a sign of Liver qi stagnation as well, as is the case with women prone to PMS.

Even those not familiar with the five elements will have no trouble associating the element wood with intimacy and sexuality. Think about it— what's the name for an erect penis? A woodie! The clitoris also becomes erect by engorging with blood, and I liken it to a bud sprouting on a branch.

Wood-Balancing Choices: Cleansing the Body

ALCOHOL: It's romantic to watch the sunset with our beloved, toasting each other with a glass of wine—or two or three. It's sexy, relaxing, and warming to drink as a prelude to sex. But here's the question: since the liver needs to process all this alcohol-infused intimacy, does drinking help or hinder the baby-making process?

For most couples, a glass of wine once in a while is fine. How much is too much? The jury's still out on that question, but most experts say abstinence is the best policy when trying to conceive. Why? Because so often a little turns into a lot. And too much alcohol is not only bad for sperm, it can also kill sex drive. Too much beer, for example, actually decreases a man's libido, thanks to hops, its main ingredient. Drinking too much of anything alcoholic, or taking certain drugs for that matter, has been directly linked to erectile dysfunction (ED), according to the Mayo Clinic.[7] And if you are taking fertility drugs it's even more important that you avoid alcohol. Your liver is already working overtime to process the drugs and the extra hormones. The last thing it needs is to be burdened with more things to detoxify.

CAFFEINE: But surely coffee is okay, right? How about yerba maté or a big cup of Japanese matcha? Don't worry, no one is suggesting you give up your morning cuppa. In fact, many experts agree that one or two cups (300–600 mg) of your favorite morning beverage are fine and shouldn't impact your ability to conceive. The American College of Obstetrics and Gynecology suggests limiting your intake to twelve ounces of the caffeine beverage of your choice. According to my mentor, Chinese medicine and fertility expert Randine Lewis, caffeine is a central nervous system stimulant, with volatile oils that may not be that good for fertility, even when drinking a decaffeinated brew, so it's to be avoided if possible. A 2016 study by the National Institutes of Health shows a connection between miscarriage and drinking more than two caffeinated beverages a day.[8]

So much depends on how you process caffeine and what your anxiety levels are. Here's what I think: It's important to pay attention to how you feel when you're caffeinated. Some of my patients suffer from anxiety that is made worse the longer they struggle with infertility issues. For these folks I usually recommend either eliminating caffeine or switching to a cup of green tea. Most green and white teas have much less caffeine and more antioxidant properties, and antioxidants help temper the oxidative stress often associated infertility.

LIVER CLEANSING: Among the liver's many functions is regulating sex-hormone levels by eliminating any excess. If you've been undergoing assisted reproductive therapy and have been given hormones, your liver's been working overtime. So at the end of a medicated fertility cycle I encourage my patients to do a mild liver cleanse for seven to ten days. You'll find many ways to do this: most involve giving up wheat, sugar, dairy, caffeine, and alcohol, and restricting foods that could be inflammatory such as peanuts, eggs, red meat, and strawberries. I also recommend acupuncture treatments and taking specific herbs and vitamins. Confer with your acupuncturist, naturopath, osteopath, or functional medicine doctor for more detailed and personalized advice.

Wood Element Emotion: Sexual Frustration

Sexual frustration can be described as pent-up energy needing release, which can happen to one or both partners in a relationship so focused on baby-making. The best way to move that stuck energy is to commit to loving and honest communication—owning your feelings and expressing them in a nonblaming, nonjudgmental way, and finding little ways of connecting sensually that go beyond sexual pleasure. We are designed to take in the beauty that's all around us: in nature, music, animals, chance connections, food, spirituality, and yes, sex. Love is that state of being where we remember that there is no separation between where I end and you begin; we see the Divine in ourselves and in the other. Put aside all the rules you've adhered to about lovemaking and focus on pleasure. Don't be afraid to ask for what you need, and be sure to ask your beloved the question "How can I love you more?"

THE WATER ELEMENT: REPRODUCTIVE ENERGY

The water element constitutes the deepest aspect of our being because this element involves reproductive energy—our sexuality. In Chinese medicine, Kidney and Bladder qi, which correlate with the adrenal glands that sit atop the kidneys in Western anatomy, comprise the water element in the body.

Will and determination, two characteristics of the water element, drive your desire to make a baby—and you need that. However, if you focus solely on your resolve and don't temper it with patience and generosity, you can burn out. Western doctors say that burnout results in adrenal fatigue; Chinese medicine says this in terms of depleted jing—our vital Kidney energy. No matter how it's described, it all translates to plummeting sex drive and no baby. Taoists say the antidote to burnout is to find the middle path and commit to a life of balance between yin and yang, being and doing.

The water element contains fire energy as well, what Taoists call the "minister fire." Think of Kidney energy as the pilot light for the furnace that ignites our vital energies. When the fire is strong, we enjoy a healthy, strong sex drive. When it's flickering or diminished . . . well, my patient Jenny is a good example of what happens.

Jenny is an exercise junkie. She took spinning class five times a week, worked out with weights three times a week, and got in a ten-mile run on the weekends. To do all that and hold down a job, she had to get up at five in the morning. By the time she made her way home at the end of her day she was pretty much wiped out and had no energy left for intimacy. When she first started seeing me she was completely exhausted, although *she* couldn't see that. The dark circles under her eyes signaled weak Kidney qi and low cortisol (adrenal fatigue). She needed to replenish her minister fire and give her body a much-needed rest. She agreed to cut back on exercise, find more time to relax with her husband and see more of their friends, and commit to acupuncture and nutritional supplements to reset her nervous system and build her reserves back up. Changing her regimen actually helped her feel more "in her body," more sensual, and her sex drive increased dramatically.

To keep the water element flowing, commit to activities that help decrease stress—rest, walking in nature, and mindful exercise such as yoga and qigong are all great for alleviating stress; meditation is, of course, highly beneficial, as are massage and acupuncture.

Water Element: Kidney Energy Tonics

Classic Chinese medicine texts include herbal medicine among the ways to rebuild Kidney energy, which can translate into healthy libido and, hopefully, successful reproduction. Here are a few of the more popular herbs practitioners suggest. Of course, it's always advisable to talk with a Chinese medicine specialist who can offer recommendations tailored to your individual challenges. Note that most Chinese herbs are taken together as formulas as opposed to individually.

HORNY GOAT WEED (*Epimedium* spp., yin yang huo): A leafy plant native to Asia and the Mediterranean, this hormone regulator is often added to formulas that increase Kidney yang energy, improve libido, and treat erectile dysfunction. With a name like horny goat weed, it'd be hard to pass up. Some studies suggest this herb helps with immune function, depression, and bone health. The usual dose is 500 mg two to three times a day. Caution: don't use if you have low blood pressure.

REHMANNIA (*Rehmannia glutinosa*, Chinese foxglove, shu di huang, sheng di huang): This Chinese herb of restoration, a chief ingredient in most Kidney energy supplements, is said to nourish the blood, address anemia, and help Kidney yin. In Western medicine, rehmannia is an adrenal tonic that focuses on exhaustion, menstrual disorders, and hormonal dysfunction. While not an aphrodisiac per se, balancing hormone function often improves sex drive. Take rehmannia as part of an herbal formula containing other herbs.

CORDYCEPS (*Cordyceps* spp.): A type of fungus originally found on the backs of caterpillars in the Himalayas, *Cordyceps* is a genus that includes some four hundred species and is now grown in laboratories. A prized herb in Chinese medicine, cordyceps enhances cellular energy, increases sperm count, normalizes immune function, enhances athletic performance, replenishes normal energy stores, and increases sexual function. The usual dose is about 500 to 1000 mg a day.

MACA (*Lepidium meyenii*, Peruvian ginseng): Grown in the Andes in Peru, this root has been shown to have a beneficial effect not only on libido, but also on sperm count and motility. It is considered an adaptogen, a class of herbs that stabilizes physiological processes and promotes homeostasis. Thirteen types of maca exist, each with a different function. The three most popular types for fertility are black maca, yellow maca, and red maca. Black maca appears to have better effects on sperm production than its yellow cousin, and red maca seems to reduce prostate size and is good for women's libidos. Yellow maca is geared to improving adrenal function and men's sexual health. Choosing the right product makes a big difference in the outcome, so check with a Chinese medicine specialist or an herbalist familiar with this root.

ASHWAGANDHA (*Withania somnifera*, Indian ginseng): This Ayurvedic adaptogenic herb helps the body resist the damaging inflammatory effects of stress and calms the nervous system. Ashwagandha has performed well in studies, substantially reducing serum cortisol levels with mild, if any, side effects and improving sperm overall.[9] We already know how stress can dampen libido, so ashwagandha deserves its place on the libido-enhancing top-ten list. To cement its reputation, ashwagandha can be used as an aphrodisiac.

MUIRA PUAMA (*Ptychopetalum* spp., potency wood): This herb, harvested from a small tree in the Amazon, is said to improve erectile dysfunction and increase libido. A small study found that the combination of ginkgo biloba and muira puama can significantly improve sexual desire and frequency of sexual intercourse in women.[10] Participants reported increased satisfaction with their sex life, intensity of sexual desires and fantasies, an easier time reaching orgasm, and intensity of orgasm. Dosage is typically 1000 to 1500 mg of a 4-to-1 extract.

Water Element Emotion: Fear

The dream of having a child is the longing of the heart to experience love, to nurture, and to create. For many women struggling with fertility, fear is a constant companion. *What if I never get pregnant? I have to have a baby by the age of forty or my life is over.* Doctors aren't always very sensitive to the fear factor in women trying to conceive and often exacerbate it by reciting a litany of factors on why conception may never happen, such as age, weight, and stress. Of course, fear can get in the way of the body's ability to conceive because it messes with the nervous system's balance, putting it into fight-flight-freeze mode, effectively shutting down the reproductive system (chapter 12 has many helpful ideas for countering fear). The antidote to fear is any practice that keeps you in the present, any practice that focuses on love, patience, compassion, and forgiveness. Certainly acknowledging your fear—and the reasons for it—can help. Allow yourself to be held; practice self-love, and take deep, gentle, healing breaths, saying over and over again "I see you, I love you, you are whole, you are enough." And practice gratitude.

THE FIRE ELEMENT: AWAKENING TO THE SPIRIT OF JOY AND LOVE

Summer governs the fire element. We want to stay out later, play, have fun, be in the sun. Summer is the most yang time of the year, which means we have more energy and desire to connect outwardly and let love in (as well, see chapter 8). In Chinese medicine, fire energy is associated with Heart and Small Intestine, the Pericardium, and what's known as the "Triple Burner" (corresponding to the three different areas of the abdomen: upper, middle, and lower, and related to the movement of water). If your fire energy is weak, you may feel depressed, uninspired, and unable to show your vulnerabilities. In the bedroom, a weak fire element translates to a lack of passion, the feeling that you're just going through the motions without any heart in it.

Conversely, raging fire energies can leave you feel overwhelmed and out of control. As a result, sometimes men feel the need to masturbate and ejaculate two to three times a day to relieve the stress. That can be a problem for baby-making sex because excessive masturbation wastes precious seed, especially around the fertile window. Remember that the kidneys rely on a steady pilot light to keep our vital energy, our sexuality, burning bright. When the fire of the Kidney energy rages, it abandons its correct place and blazes upward to the heart, depleting a man's vital essence. To enjoy optimal health and strong libido, the fire in the heart must be in balance with the water energy of the kidneys. When the fire element is in tune, we sleep soundly, have more fun, and love more deeply. (More tips in chapter 8.)

Fire Element Tonics

In Chinese medicine, daytime is active or yang in nature, and nighttime is quiet or yin in nature. We must have a balance of the two to be healthy. One of the ways we sabotage our fertility is by not getting enough sleep. Yaron Seidman, a Chinese medicine doctor and the author of *Curing Infertility: The Incredible Hunyuan Breakthrough* told me, "When we sleep, we recharge, and recharging keeps our youth and our fertility."[11] The best sleep comes, Seidman explains, when we synchronize our schedule with nature. That means in wintertime, when nights are long, we should go to bed at 10 p.m., and in summertime, when the sun sets much later, we can extend that to 11 p.m.

"Being too tired is the #1 reason women blame for their loss of desire,"[12] according to Laurie Mintz, PhD, an expert on the psychology of human sexuality and the author of *A Tired Woman's Guide to Passionate Sex*. Obviously, the solution is to add more zzzz's to your life—the good-quality kind. Men, too. Research suggests that too little sleep can lower testosterone levels. So do what you need to do—go to bed earlier to recharge your energy and actually have time for intimacy even if it's in the morning. Yoga nidra, a deeply restorative practice (described in chapter 12), can help. Practice it for fifteen or twenty minutes at least two hours before you're ready to head off to sleep. Once in bed, try progressive relaxation techniques to calm body and mind. As well, a couple of promising studies suggest that supplementing with melatonin may help with fertility problems.[13]

EXERCISE: Being physically fit is an asset for conception and sexuality. But, as my patient Jenny discovered, too much of a good thing is never a good thing, and that is the case with exercise. Studies show that too much exercise (more than sixty minutes a day) can cause some women to stop ovulating—a condition called "anovulation"—and that vigorous exercise for thirty to sixty minutes a day is associated with a reduced risk of anovulatory infertility.[14] Of course, the key is balance. In a cross-section survey of 1,077 men published in *Medicine and Science in Sports and Exercise*, researchers concluded that endurance training at high levels of intensity for longer periods of time on a regular basis is "significantly associated with decreased libido scores in men."[15] Researchers noted that therapists who treat male patients for sexual disorders or who counsel couples on infertility issues should consider the level of endurance exercise of one or both partners as a potential complicating factor. Though the emphasis in that study was on overdoing things, another 2017 study of infertile males between the ages of twenty-five and forty found that 24 weeks of moderate aerobic exercise favorably helped with semen markers of inflammation and oxidative stress.[16]

Getting the picture? Moderate exercise such as yoga, pilates, cross-training, swimming, walking, hiking, dancing, biking (in moderation—sitting in the saddle for too long can negatively impact sperm production as can too much exercise) is great for conception. As an exercise physiologist myself, I often recommend exercise to increase strength, endurance, and flexibility, as well as to relieve stress and help increase endorphins, those feel-good chemicals your body produces. Caution: If you are doing assisted reproductive medicine, make sure you follow your doctor's guidelines regarding exercise.

CONNECT TO YOUR HIGHER POWER: As described in chapter 4, the spirit of fire is shen, our spiritual energy or enlightened awareness—one of the Three Treasures of Chinese medicine. Heart shen is the universal love that connects us all. It reminds us to bring our hearts together when we make love. When you open your heart up to love, the energy flows up the body to your heart and out through the crown. Connecting to your heart allows you to trust your spiritual journey of procreation, even when it is fraught with uncertainty, even when you have no idea whether you will ever have a child. Shen reminds you to love more, laugh more, and bring more joy into your life. When you have ample shen, you have *joie de vivre*—a love of life, a sense of purpose. Your body feels strong, your mind is clear, and your heart is full. When shen, the element of fire, dims, you may feel discouraged, restless, and inadequate. On the most basic level, the emotion of a balanced fire element is joy.

YOGA: This holistic mind-body practice can be quite helpful for enhancing desire and encouraging a more loving connection with your partner. A few caveats, however. Stay away from Hot Yoga or any yoga practice where the room is heated above 90 degrees, because excessive heat can dry up the body's fluids—what in Chinese medicine is the yin energy you need to make a baby. Hala Khori, a longtime yoga teacher and a practitioner of Peter Levine's Somatic Experiencing (see chapter 11), says that the benefits of yoga extend far beyond promoting flexibility and strength. "Yoga is learning to be with discomfort without running away," she says. "We often get into uncomfortable poses and we are asked to simply breathe and be present with our discomfort." She recommends that you find a yoga practice that feels safe, healing, and healthy for you. Notice what you are drawn to. She explains that "type A people might need to move or flow a little in order to get still, and a class that allows for this is a good fit. If it's just movement and no stillness, you never get to settle. Then there are people who are drawn to yin or other, more meditative styles. They may need to move a little so they don't perpetuate their imbalance."

If you don't live in a city that offers yoga for fertility, you can always supplement with a home practice (see the resources section at the back of this book).

When we attend to our body, mind, and heart, we become present to who we really are and conscious of the life-giving energy that resides in every cell—an energy that needs our care and nourishment. When we attend to ourselves we maximize our capacity to experience love. Baby-making is an opportunity to not only pay attention to our own needs, but to also connect and share that experience with our partner. This allows us to feel more deeply, experience more pleasure, and hopefully have fun in the process. And sure, there will be moments of discomfort, but there is always a return to love, to the energy of the heart. That is where conception lives—in the vast ocean of love.

SEXUAL SECRET
Taoist Position to Balance the Five Elements and Strengthen Bone Marrow

Have the woman lie facedown with a pillow under her belly. Make sure she is well-lubricated and aroused. Gentlemen, enter from the rear and give seventy-two thrusts of love with your jade stalk. Not sure how to do thrusts? Try this Taoist secret in any position. Start with nine shallow thrusts and then give one deep one. Next, give eight shallow strokes and two deep ones, then seven shallow strokes and three deep ones. Continue on until you reach ten deep ones. Don't worry if you lose count. This is a recipe for healing and pleasure.

The Five-Element
Lover's Wheel

....

IN CHINESE MEDICINE, we use the five elements, also called the five phases, of nature—wood, fire, earth, metal, and water—to diagnose and treat individuals. Native Americans also use circles in the form of medicine wheels. Stones placed in the center, embodying the four directions, also have a special symbolism for health and healing. Normally, the five elements are arranged in a circle showing there is no beginning and no end and that the elements must live in harmony with each other.

I've created two five-element wheels based on the five elements of Chinese medicine. These wheels provide a visual shorthand for how each element presents when it's in balance and when it's out of balance. I have used the ancient Taoist diagram of the five elements that puts the earth element in the center. After all, the earth is the fertile ground where life grows. With earth as the center of our being, Taoists believe that yang sheng—the practice of nurturing and nourishing life—increases health and longevity. Modern Chinese medicine practitioners would say the same is true for fertility. To live a life of balance we must live in harmony with all five elements of nature.

Gina Ogden, an award-winning sex therapist and teacher, created "the four-dimensional wheel of sexual experience," which includes physical, emotional, mental, and spiritual aspects of sexuality. Inspired by her work, I incorporated sexuality into the Chinese medicine five element model.

Working with these lover's wheels invites you to see which of the five elements you most resonate with right now and which of the five elements may need more attention. All five elements are interdependent, each one sustaining and nurturing the others, such that the health of one depends on the health of the others—much like the chakra system in yoga. For example, communication (the earth element) helps us express our fantasies, needs, and desires (wood element) so that we can satisfy our animal nature (metal element). However, if there are imbalances in the elements—if we don't feel desirable (earth element), if we have past hurts and traumas that wrap parts of our body in armor (metal element), or if we are scared and don't fully trust our partner (water element), we will have nothing to communicate except perhaps the pain of separation and a feeling of emptiness.

Use these elements as a tool of inquiry to allow you to see where you might need some extra attention. For example, when I met my new partner years after my husband passed away, I would cry every time we made love. I understood that this was grief (metal element out of balance) still held in my body. Luckily, my partner understood. He was patient with me, allowing my body to de-armor and open at its own pace. We breathed a lot together (metal element in balance).

Look to see what element or elements command your attention. Are you always trying to please your partner but not asking for what you want (earth element out of balance)? Do you feel angry at your partner, preventing you from wanting to make love (wood energy out of balance), and what would correct communication (earth energy in balance) and get back to love (fire energy in balance)?

THE FIVE-ELEMENT LOVER'S WHEEL: IN BALANCE

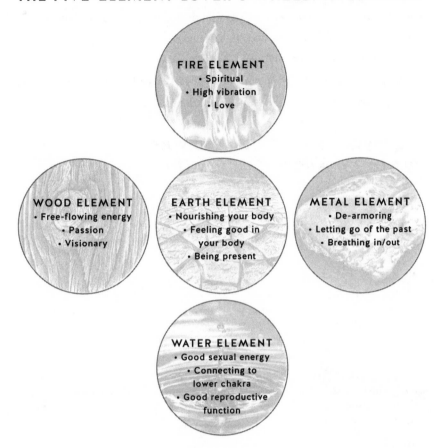

A Balanced Relationship to All That Is

THE EARTH ELEMENT: Nourishing your body helps you feel good physically, which allows you to make love with full attention and devotion. When you connect willingly, you merge with your beloved and raise your own vibration and that of the planet.

THE METAL ELEMENT: Balanced metal allows you to be fully present, opening places within that have shut down and releasing past disappointments and heartache by focusing on the breath.

THE WATER ELEMENT: Releasing stress through meditation, a balancing yoga or qigong practice, and appropriate herbs and supplements enhances sexual energy and reproductive function.

THE WOOD ELEMENT: Balanced wood invites you to flow with whatever life presents. It ignites your passion and gives you permission to be a sexual adventurer along with your partner.

THE FIRE ELEMENT: Balanced fire keeps your vital energy burning brightly, with more desire to connect outwardly and an openness to love. You sleep soundly, have more fun, and love more deeply.

THE FIVE-ELEMENT LOVER'S WHEEL: OUT OF BALANCE

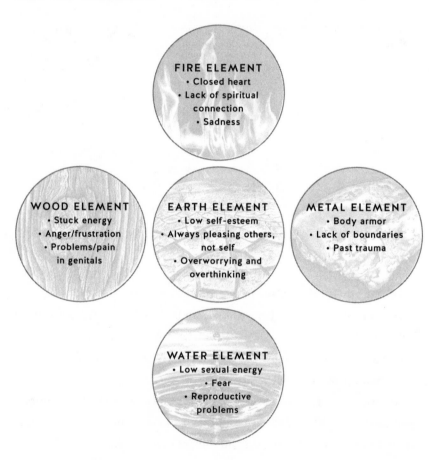

An Out-of-Balance Relationship to All That Is

THE EARTH ELEMENT: You've lost your center and your self-confidence. Excessive worrying and preoccupation with what your partner thinks make it hard to open your heart to experience the spiritual/heart connection in your relationship.

THE METAL ELEMENT: Unbalanced metal is often caused by unresolved sexual trauma, which keeps you shut down. It can also mean you don't know how to establish boundaries, oftentimes saying "yes" when you really mean "no."

THE WATER ELEMENT: Unbalanced water manifests as exhaustion, low libido, and fear, resulting in an unbalanced nervous system and reproductive difficulties.

THE WOOD ELEMENT: Unbalanced wood gives rise to sexual frustration and often manifests physically as genital pain or other difficulties in the sex organs.

THE FIRE ELEMENT: Unbalanced fire produces a lack of passion, a sense of simply going through the motions. It can cause depression, a "what's the use" attitude, and feeling disconnected from your spiritual side.

Now that you've been introduced to the five elements of Chinese medicine and how they fit on the wheel of sexual energy, you are ready to identify where you sit on the wheel in terms of one or possibly more elements. The following exercises will assist you in determining what's out of balance; you can then use the suggested practices and acupressure points on yourself and your partner to help strengthen those elements that need strengthening.

Investigating your relationship to each element can help you discover where you're blocked and what you need to do to create more balance in your body, mind, and spirit. The first exercise will help you get started; you may want to do it alone the first time, and then try it with your partner, sharing your findings with each other. It's a great way to initiate or deepen the conversation without inviting defensiveness or justifications.

Each exercise in this chapter includes specific questions, practices, and some acupressure points that you can press on yourself or on each other to strengthen the element in question. Though for each element I have chosen only a few points to press, there are so many more possibilities to choose from, so be sure to check the resources section at the end of this book for more ideas.

A word on acupuncture/acupressure points: These points have their own measurements, called *cun*; 1 cun is equal the the width of your thumb; 1.5 cun equals the width of your index and middle finger; 2 cun is the measurement from the tip of the index finger to the crease of second knuckle; and 3 cun is equal to the width of all four fingers. In case this all sounds too complicated, I've tried to locate the area using anatomical landmarks. But really, if you go to the general area, you are bound to find the right point.

Most acupressure points call for pressing or rubbing for four to ten seconds, or tapping three to six times. Many points will feel achy or tender when stimulated. Pay attention to what feels good to you and what feels good to your partner; in other words, always ask for, and listen to, feedback.

THE PRACTICE

First, take a piece of paper and write down where on the wheel you self-identify and where on the wheel you see your partner. Second, answer the questions posed for those "spokes." Third, do the exercises associated with them, and finally, share the results with your partner, if you wish.

EARTH ELEMENT: THE DEVOTED LOVER
Earth Essence: Communication

You set your intention by planting a seed in the ground; you water it with your love and your actions, which helps it bear fruit. Declare your devotion to yourself and to your beloved so that you both feel secure and the relationship can stand on solid ground. Communicate how you want to be cared for, how you want to be touched, and what your needs and desires are in order to connect sexually.

The Key to Earth Energy

Nourish yourself by first finding your own center, and then nourish your relationship. You want to take care of yourself so you have enough energy to feel love and to truly make love. As an earth-centered being, strive to feel comfortable in your body, without judgmental thoughts like *I am too fat, my breasts are too small, I am not enough.*

Earth Questions

How often does your mind wander during lovemaking?

How easy is it for you ask for what you want sexually?

Do you ever find yourself saying "yes" to things when you really mean "no," in order to please your partner—and then becoming resentful?

Do you often have a difficult time finding your own voice and setting boundaries?

What is your relationship with your body? How do you feel about your partner's body?

EARTH PRACTICE

The Mirror Exercise

Stand in front of a full-length mirror naked. Allow yourself to see the beauty that is you. Revel in the curves, size, and shape of all the areas of your body, including your vulva (or penis). Focus on an area that you actually admire in your body—everyone has at least one. Rub your hands over your body. Feel yourself; caress your body. Notice what comes up for you as you consciously affirm your love for yourself. Do this every day.

Earth Acupressure Points

For each one, press or rub for four to ten seconds using medium pressure.

STOMACH 36 (ST 36)–ZU SAN LI, "LEG THREE MILES": This is an important point for strengthening and enriching the body, mind, and spirit. Used to relieve fatigue.

Location: Four finger-widths (3 cun) down from the bottom of your knee-cap, along the outer border of your shinbone. The point should feel a little achy when pressed, so fish around until you feel the tenderness (see figure 1 at the end of the chapter).

REN 6/CONCEPTION VESSEL 6 (CV 6)–QI HAI, "SEA OF QI": This point is used to tap into the deeper reserves of energy to increase sexual vitality.

Location: Place your index and middle finger together horizontally and place them directly below your belly button (1.5 cun). The point is located just below your middle finger underneath your belly button (see figure 2).

SPLEEN 4 (SP 4)–GONG SUN, "GRANDFATHER GRANDSON": This is the opening point or master point for the Chong Mai vessel, which is connected to your sex organs (more on this in chapter 11). When you want to tell your body that you are going to use this vessel, begin by pressing this point.

Location: Start at your big toe and slide your hand up the inside of the big toe to the first metatarsal, the long bone in the foot, the part closest to the heel. The point is in a depression in the long bone where the red skin (bottom of foot) and white skin (top of foot) meet (see figure 3).

METAL ELEMENT: YOUR ANIMAL NATURE
Metal Essence: Engaging the Body and Senses

The metal element invites you to let go of the past and connect with your animal nature—not always easy, especially for women. This energy is the spirit of the metal element, which Taoists call *po.* In lovemaking, you must commit to being fully present in your body, fully engaged with your senses, and fully present to your lover. The energy of the element metal invites you to let go of past hurts, traumas, and any unresolved psychological issues so that you can carry out your vision, which comes from the wood element. To do that, you must commit to healing your mind and body through the somatic practices of acupuncture/acupressure; this will bring the memories stored within your body that are not consciously received by your mind into the light of awareness. You cannot fully open to your sexuality without healing any separation between your body and your mind. When you do begin to heal, you will open a door to exploring and celebrating your sexual self. That might mean you want to explore fantasy, a form of play expressed by the wood element.

The Key to Metal Energy

The breath connects you to the element of metal. It's almost impossible to be fully present in your own body and with your lover when you're stressed or anxious. Simple breathing practices can help you release tension and stress so that you can show up fully.

Metal Questions

Are you holding on to grief and not allowing yourself to feel?

What do you need to get rid of that no longer serves you or that gets in the way of being fully present in your body—old memories, stuck emotions or ideas?

Where do you hold all of that stuckness in your body?

METAL PRACTICES

Qigong Shaking Exercise

Shaking helps move energy. Stand with your feet hip-width apart, knees slightly bent, arms at your sides. Feel your feet rooted in the earth, as if you are a tree. Keeping your shoulders soft, begin bouncing your whole body. Shake all over, including your legs and arms. Shake loose anything you're holding on to. Shake to your own rhythm. Add some music if you like—there's really no right or wrong way to shake. Feel your animal nature. Don't be surprised if sounds start to come out of your mouth as you begin to let go. You can practice this as often as you like—anywhere from two minutes to twenty minutes a day.

continues

TCM Exercise to Move Stuck Emotions

To begin, take a few full breaths, inhaling through your nose and exhaling through your mouth. On your next inhalation, visualize a healing white light entering your body from the top of your head, at your crown; as you exhale, make the sound *sssss* (the sound of a snake), releasing any emotions stored in your body.

Alternate-Nostril Breath

A breathing technique from yoga, *nadi shodhana*, or alternate-nostril breath, helps balance the nervous system. The left nostril is associated with yin and is calming, while the right nostril is associated with yang and is activating.

1. Find a comfortable seated position. Brenda Strong, creator of Strong Yoga®4Women, a program for increasing fertility, suggests sitting on the floor with a soft fertility ball she has created placed at the acupuncture point Ren 1 (between the anus and the back of the labia majora) for not more than two minutes; or you can sit with one leg outstretched and place the heel of the other foot at acupuncture point Ren 1.
2. Begin by taking a few deep breaths.
3. Use the thumb of the right hand to close the right nostril and gently and fully inhale through the left nostril.
4. Close the left nostril with the fourth finger of the right hand, release your thumb from your right nostril, and exhale through the right nostril.
5. Keeping the left nostril closed, begin to inhale through the right nostril.
6. Close the right nostril with the thumb, release your fourth finger from your left nostril, and exhale through the left nostril. This is one full round.
7. Repeat these steps for ten full rounds.

Metal Element: Acupressure Points

Rub or tap each point for four to ten seconds with medium pressure.

LUNG 1 (LU 1)–ZHONG FU, "MIDDLE PALACE": This point is helpful for those who are grief-stricken, to help them connect with heavenly qi and inspiration—and a great place to caress on the way to the breasts. (See figure 2.)

Location: Starting on the side of the upper chest, in line with the first intercostal space (between the ribs), 6 cun (eight finger breadths) from the center of the chest. In this area where the shoulder meets the chest, you'll feel a large hollow known as the deltopectoral triangle, just under the outer third of the collarbone. The point is located about a thumb's width beneath this clavicle.

LUNG 7 (LU 7)–LIE QUE, "NARROW DEFILE": This is an opening point for Ren Mai (the Conception Vessel), which connects to the uterus. It's a good point if you are holding tension around the shoulders and chest and have constricted breathing.

Location: About two finger breadths (the index and middle finger, or 1.5 cun) above the wrist crease and in line with the thumb between its two tendons. For anatomy geeks this means the brachioradialis and abductor pollicis (see figure 4).

URINARY BLADDER 42 (UB 42)–PO HU, "SOUL DOOR": Located on the back, this point corresponds to the lungs. UB 42 connects with the spiritual aspect of the lungs, the po, and to your animal nature and your breath. This point can revive the spirit if there is grief or long-term sadness.

Location: On the back on the border of the scapula in line with the third thoracic vertebrae, about four fingers away from the midline (3 cun) (see figure 5).

WATER ELEMENT: DESIRE

Water Essence: Primal Desire/Sexual Fulfillment

The energy created by water is the life force that flows through every cell, muscle, joint, and channel in your body. It is your primal sexual energy, which lives in the second chakra. This energy represents the aspect of yourself that longs for deep sexual fulfillment and union with your beloved. It asks you to trust your instinctual reproductive nature and to not fear that time is running out.

By focusing on the water element you can feel into your sex drive and cultivate it. It's the lustful feeling of being turned-on, being praised, being desired—and desiring your beloved. Kidney energy, which is governed by the element water, opens all the way to the ears, so water essence encourages you to listen to what your partner has to say.

The Key to Water Energy

The water element is concentrated in the kidneys. Connecting your sexual life force (Kidney qi) with the energy of your heart and merging it with that of your beloved is the energy of making a baby. There is no separation.

Water Questions

The water element asks you to examine the unknown; what are the hidden, fearful, or insecure parts of yourself?

What keeps you from intimacy?

What are you afraid of?

What gets in the way of fully participating in lovemaking?

What keeps you from truly hearing your beloved?

WATER PRACTICE

Partner yoga enhances fertility and increases sexuality.

Passing the Ball

Brenda Strong shares this practice for partners that she created for her Strong Yoga®4Women program.

1. Lean with your backs against each other while you both sit in a comfortable cross-legged position. Take a moment to feel the support of your partner's back against yours. On the back is the acupuncture point UB 23 (see figure 5 for exact location), which gets stimulated in this position.
2. Begin to use *ujjayi* yoga breathing, also known as "ocean breath." To do this, close your lips, rest the tip of your tongue behind your front teeth, and breathe in and out of your nose. Next, inhale through your nose and constrict the muscles in the back of your throat. Exhale and continue to constrict your throat muscles as if making the sound *haaaah*, but with your lips closed.
3. Both partners place their hands in a downward-facing triangle just below the belly button, the second chakra, which is the seat of creation, the place where the sexual organs are housed.

4. Partner A: Inhale through the nose, filling your belly, allowing your hands to rise with your belly, as if you are filling the shape of a pregnant belly. Then, as you exhale through your nose, lightly press your hands into your belly as it deflates.

5. Partner B: As Partner A exhales, you begin to inhale through your nose, bringing your attention to your hands and expanding your belly outward as if you are filling an energy ball that has been passed to you from your partner.

6. Partner B: Exhale through your nose as you gently press your hands into your belly, deflating your belly and passing the energy ball to your partner.

7. Partner A: As your partner exhales, you repeat step 5.

Continue to pass the energy ball back and forth between the two of you through the second chakra, breathing together like a continuous wave. This practice Brenda told me "is very sensual, intimate, and exciting because you can feel the heat increase in your low back as you pass this energy ball between the two of you. It gets the juices flowing without any words needing to be said." It's a beautiful way to "develop a sense of connection . . . intimacy and charge within the sexual center."

Water Acupuncture Points

Rub the following points for four to ten seconds using medium pressure.

KIDNEY 7 (KID 7)–FU LIU, "RETURNING CURRENT": This is a nourishing point for Kidney energy, beneficial for reproduction and sexual functioning.

Location: Beginning at the space between the anklebone (tip of the medial malleolus) and the achilles tendon, moving 2 cun above that point (see figure 3).

REN 4/CONCEPTION VESSEL 4 (CV 4)–GUAN YUAN, "FIRST GATE": This point nourishes and strengthens the whole system, including your sex drive, and fortifies Kidney jing for conception and birth. If you cruise downward from this point you will connect with Ren 2 (above the pubic bone) to heighten more arousal. In fact, the whole line between the belly button and the pubic bone is great to massage.

Location: Directly above the pubic bone, using the tip of your index finger to the crease of the second knuckle (2 cun) (see figure 2).

URINARY BLADDER 23 (UB 23)–SHEN SHU, "KIDNEY CORRESPONDENCE": This point nourishes Kidney essence, stoking the fire when you lack desire or have fertility challenges.

Location: on the lower back, two fingers wide (1.5 cun), lateral to the lower border of the spinous process of the second lumbar vertebra (see figure 5).

WOOD ELEMENT: VISIONARY
Wood Essence: Passion and Dreams

The wood element supports your passions and dreams. Maybe you've always wanted to make love on a boat. Maybe your lover's fantasy is to dress up and role-play. To become a more passionate lover, your wood energy needs to flow freely. As the energy moves unencumbered, your lovemaking can carry out your vision for baby-making. When the wood element is balanced, you are not bogged down by unprocessed emotions that you can't express such as anger, sadness, or frustration, all of which can get in the way of lovemaking. Movement can help you free stuck energy and so can trying different sexual positions. You need ample wood to make a fire.

The Key to Wood

You connect to this element through the eyes and eye-gazing.

Wood Questions

Where do you feel stuck?
Are you able to connect with your desires, dreams, and fantasies?
How does it feel to share those with your partner?

WOOD PRACTICE

Qigong Meridian Tapping

This exercise is also used as a warm-up for qigong practice. It's like an acupressure massage with an invigorating quality. We include it in the wood element, but it really moves energy on all the meridians throughout the body.

Begin by standing with feet hip-width apart and knees slightly bent. Use the palms of your hands or the pads of your four fingers, gently cupping them and tapping up and down the energy pathways.

Order of tapping: first invigorate the upper body and then the lower body.

1. Raise your right arm; tap under the armpit and down the side of the body around to the belly button and up the midline.
2. Tap down the top of your right shoulder along the outside of the arm to the top of the hand.
3. Turn your hand over and tap on the inside of the hand up the inside of the arm to your right shoulder.
4. Repeat this sequence on your left side.
5. Bring your hands to your lower back and gently begin to tap the kidneys.
6. Continue to tap down the outside of your legs with your exhalation, down to your feet.
7. Then tap with your inhalation up the inside of your legs to below your belly button.
8. Tap the Ren 6 point nine times, putting energy in your *dantien*, the "sea of qi" or energy center, located 1.5 cun below the belly button.
9. Repeat this sequence on both sides a second time.
10. Take a few full, even breaths. Your energy should be flowing now.

Wood Acupuncture Points

LIVER 3 (LV 3)–TAI CHONG, "SUPREME RUSHING": This is one of my favorite points because it helps move energy and is also related to the Chong meridian. When we combine it with LI 4 we can release tension.

Location: Between the big toe and the second toe, close to where the metatarsal (long bones of the big and second toe) meet (see figure 6).

LARGE INTESTINE 4 (LI 4)–HE GU, "JOINING VALLEY": In combination with LV 3, above, these points are called the "Four Gates" and are used to relieve intense general anxiety and many other symptoms, including headache, neck pain, and facial pain. If your partner says, "Not tonight, Honey, I have a headache," you'll know just which point to press.

Location: Between the thumb and the first finger in the middle of the webbing (see figure 4). It is a tender spot. Massage for four to five seconds. This point can contract the uterus, so don't do this if you're already pregnant.

URINARY BLADDER 18 (UB 18)–GAN SHU, "LIVER CORRESPONDENCE": This point is vital to engage when you have unprocessed emotions that feel stuck, such as anger, depression, irritability, frustration, chronic stress, or PMS. Use this point to move the stuck energy up and out of the body.

Location: On the back, 1.5 cun to the side of the thoracic vertebrae T9 (midback) (see figure 5). Have your partner rub the muscles of the back, parallel to the spine, and they'll hit it.

FIRE ELEMENT: LIGHT OF THE SPIRIT
Fire Essence: Love and Romance

You need to feel into your own heart space to access the richness of what it means to deeply love, what it means to connect as one with your partner. Heart energy embodies the slow nature of making love with intensity and great tenderness, where any distinction between you and me simply falls away—the type of unhurried lovemaking that is accessed through affection, care, emotional security, and deep, slow kissing. To open your heart to where spirit and sex meet (the water element), the fire lover must feel trust, for it is there in your heart that lies your connection to the Divine, to Spirit, and to love. It is through your heart, not your mind, that you learn to love.

The Key to Fire Energy

You connect to the element fire through your heart and through your tongue, by kissing and tasting each other.

Fire Questions

How do you define love for yourself?

What do you do to connect with your own heart?

What do you do to connect with the heart of another?

What are your spiritual beliefs and how do they impact your ability to show passion?

Do you need to practice forgiveness to be fully present in your heart?

FIRE PRACTICE

Partner Open-Heart Yoga

I like the idea of doing couples backbend yoga to open up the heart energies.

1. Person A sits in an easy cross-legged position, arms out to the sides, palms facing down.
2. Person B sits behind A, in an easy cross-legged position, facing away from A, back-to-back, connecting hearts.
3. Both partners allow their arms to hang loosely at their sides.
4. Person B leans backward as A bends forward; B will feel an opening in the chest area, while A feels a stretch in the hips.
5. If it's more comfortable, B can place hands on the tops of the thighs; A can place hands by their side to support their body.
6. Both partners: Be honest with each other. Tell your partner if the stretch is too much or not enough, and if you need them to back off or lean into the pose more. When your chest is open, feel your heart energy radiating outward.
7. Switch places.

Fire Acupressure Points

REN 17/CONCEPTION VESSEL (CV 17)–TAN ZHONG, "WITHIN THE BREAST": This point helps you connect with Spirit and access divine love. Tap it to remember to be "loving awareness," as my teacher Ram Dass says, and approach life with your heart.

Location: In the center of the chest (see figure 2).

PERICARDIUM 8 (PC 8)–LAO GONG, "PALACE OF WEARINESS": This is a fire point on a fire channel and can be used to restore vitality, especially if you feel a bit down or flatlined. Conversely, this point can also be used to quiet a restless mind that ping-pongs between two extremes.

Location: Make a fist; this point is where the tip of the middle finger touches your palm (see figure 7).

YINTANG, "HALL OF IMPRESSION": This point is the same as the third-eye point and is one of my favorites for calming the mind and accessing your inner knowing. It is also a microsystem for the heart and lungs.

Location: Between the eyebrows, at the third eye (see figure 8).

SEXUAL SECRET
For Getting Out of Your Head

This simple technique can get you out of your head and into your body, ready to receive your beloved. Sometimes it's hard to turn off the constant dripping of the thinking spigot when you're worried about your performance (*Will I get an erection? What if I don't have an orgasm?*) or still mulling over the day's events. Try tapping these acupuncture points, and with some slow, deep breaths you'll begin to move the energy out of your head and into your body. Tap each acupuncture point seven times, reciting its specific phrase silently.

Yintang (the third eye, between and just above the eyebrows): *I am present in the moment.*
Ren 17 (between the nipples): *I am love.*
Ren 4 (four fingers below the belly button): *I feel my body.*

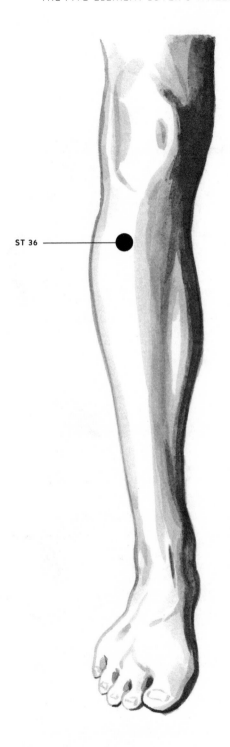

ST 36

Figure 1

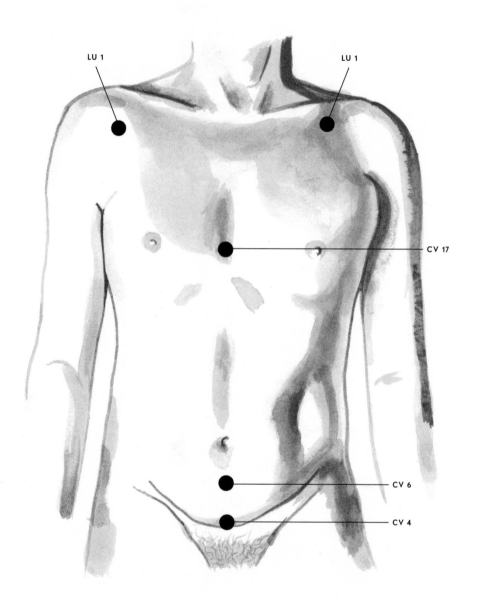

Figure 2

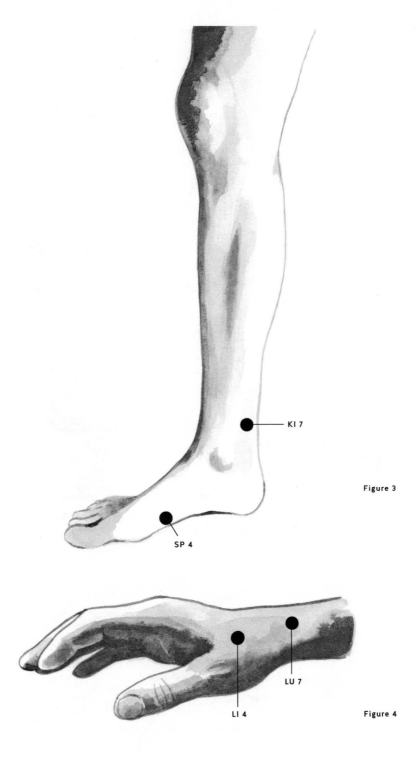

KI 7

SP 4

Figure 3

LI 4

LU 7

Figure 4

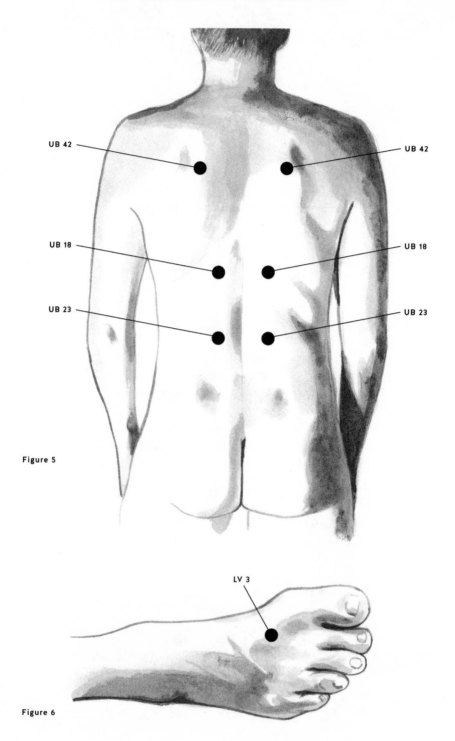

UB 42

UB 42

UB 18

UB 18

UB 23

UB 23

Figure 5

LV 3

Figure 6

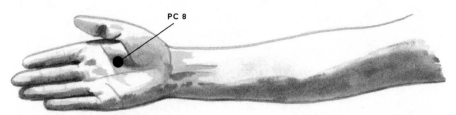

PC 8

Figure 7

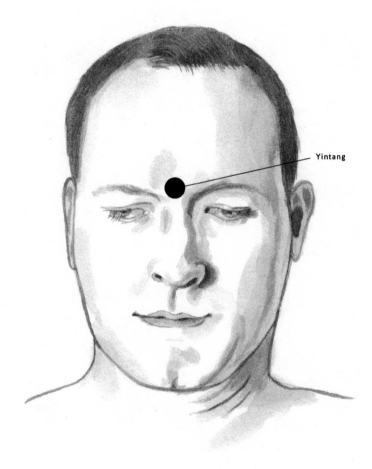

Yintang

Figure 8

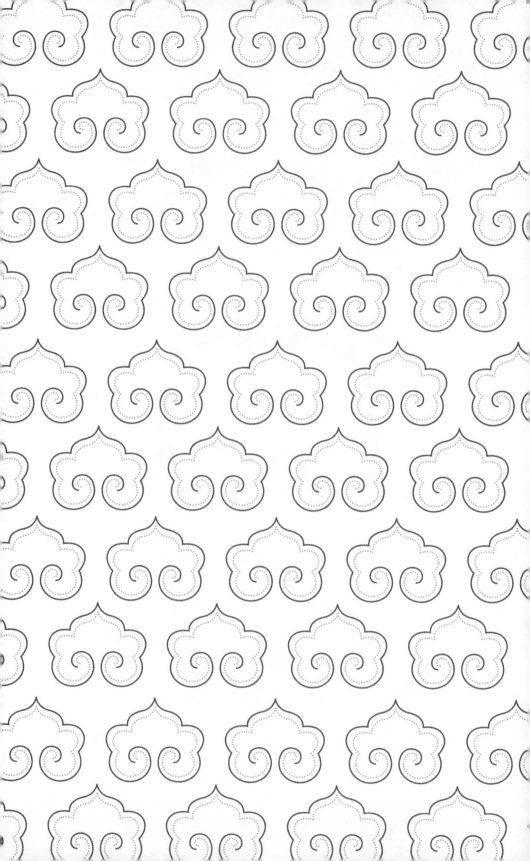

PART THREE

Creating Space

9

Fire and Flame:
Opening Up the Heart

....

Making the decision to have a child . . .
is to decide forever to have your heart
go walking outside your body.

–ELIZABETH STONE

THEY COME INTO MY OFFICE OVERWHELMED, both women and men,
not from the hours they've put in at their usual jobs, but from their "job"
of making a baby. The women pull out their phones to show me the special
apps they use to record their basal body temperature each morning before
they get out of bed. With names like Ovacue, Period Tracker, Clue, and
Fertility Friend, these apps tell women when the time is just right to call
their partners to the bedroom and get busy. Those without the app use
the old pee-on-a-stick method, where they either see one line darker than
the other or a happy face that signals "Go for it, girl!"—a cheery reminder
that they have only twelve to twenty-four hours for an egg-and-sperm
mash-up before that egg dies.

Even with all the sticks and apps, pamphlets and calendar markers,
many of the women I see still can't figure out if they're ovulating. I tell
them not to worry so much about the lines on a pee stick or basal body
temperature charts. Pay more attention to cervical mucus instead. Once
you figure out what changes to look for, you can equate those changes

with ovulation and perhaps notice an increase in your sex drive—which is what is supposed to happen biologically, right?

Unfortunately, when I say all that, the response I often get is, "*What* sex drive?" Most of these women can't even remember the last time they felt desirable or had desire. And who has time for that anyway? These women are on a mission to get sperm into their vaginas at the right time of the month. Once that's happened, they nervously wait, hopeful that they've succeeded, and, at the same time, fearful that their period will signal failure. It's almost as though they're holding their breath, getting ready for the heartbreak. As one of my patients put it, "I know if we just had sex more often my husband would feel better. I would too, but how do I get my desire back when I'm so stressed out?" The juicy ritual of lovemaking, the spontaneity they once enjoyed, has been stripped away, and the connection has become as frayed as their feelings.

The men as well come to my clinic frustrated, demoralized, and at a loss as to how to fix things. Whether they're trying to make a baby by having "productive" sex or by going the reproductive medicine route, with IVF, they see the toll it's taking on their partners. It's difficult, one of my male patients admitted, because "we no longer make love. The only sex we have anymore is timed and mechanical." He confided in me that he feels pressure to perform on demand the moment his wife announces she's ovulating. And to be honest, he says, "that doesn't always go as well as I'd like, if you know what I mean."

At this point sex becomes the all-too-common issue no one wants to talk about. In fact, so many women check the box on my intake form that says "low sex drive" that I've begun to wonder whether they had much of a sex drive to begin with. As Zoë Kors, who teaches an online course called "The Big Libido: Find Your Feminine Fire," comments, "I am astounded by how many women have no desire, no libido. Women have grown up in a culture that has no context for women's sexuality."

THE LOSS OF "SEXY"

Patricia Futia, LMFT, a Southern California relationship and sex therapist, says the majority of the patients she sees are sexless couples for a variety of reasons. One of the main reasons is the deep shame one or both partners have around expressing who they are and what they long for sexually. That shame, which can happen because of a lack of sex education, prevents them from living an authentic and genuine life. Often she needs to start with sex ed before they can get to sex therapy. She gives her patients permission to reveal themselves and reminds them over and over again that their "sexuality is foundational, and to deny it is like walking around with only one leg and one arm."[1]

It's hard enough for couples to talk about their sexual needs or admit that they feel undesirable when they're not trying to get pregnant; adding fertility challenges to the mix can be a recipe for disaster. And to make matters worse, if Western medicine is involved, the "sexy" pretty much gets stripped out of the equation. One woman came to see me initially complaining of insomnia, but eventually admitted her real concern: "It all started after I began the fertility drugs. I hate how I feel on them, even though I want so badly—no, we *both* want so badly—to have a baby. I'm having a hard time. I can't sleep. I don't want to be touched. We used to be so close, and now this whole fertility business has pulled us apart."

For these couples, what once was making love to connect heart-to-heart has become an urgent chore to conceive, devoid of pleasure. When I mention baby-making sex and how mechanical it can get, they all nod their heads in agreement. It reminds me of the old Supremes song "Where Did Our Love Go?" The expediency, urgency, and business of making a baby have replaced the love, intimacy, and sacredness of making love. When that happens, I remind couples to carry within their hearts the bigger picture. Having a baby is something that we can't control, even if we use Western reproductive medicine—and I know firsthand how crazy-making *that* can be. I tell my patients to trust that their sacred union will invite the perfect soul to enter and, in the meantime, let go of the need to control. I suggest they make a pact to enjoy each other again. Having a baby is about love, making love, being love, and surrendering to love. We spend so much time thinking, planning, organizing, waiting, and hoping, we forget to attend to and nurture the fire in our hearts and the flame in our loins.

So how do couples rekindle the spark that moved them to want to create life together in the first place? According to traditional Chinese medicine (TCM), the way to regain connection and fertility is to get your heart back in the game. And how do you do that? By unblocking the pathway in the body that links Heart energy (love) and Kidney energy (fertility) to the uterus (for women) and the "palace of sperm" (for men). That pathway, aptly called the Penetrating Vessel (Chong meridian) in Chinese medicine, is one of many such meridians we call on to restore balance to a person's system. Rekindling the spark is vital, even when a couple—whether straight or LGBTQ—chooses assisted reproduction, because for all women, creating life depends on that connection between the heart and the reproductive system.

For true lovemaking to happen and conception to result, the little pilot light located in the kidney region, called Ming-men fire, must be connected to the fire that burns in the heart region. The water element governs Kidney energy, and the fire element governs Heart energy. To understand what all this means for creating life, let's have a look at both elements individually and then see how they relate to each other along the Chong meridian.

The water element, as represented by Kidney energy, is associated with the deepest aspect of our being and governs a person's reproductive energy and sexuality. Chinese medicine believes that men have an eight-year reproductive cycle and women a seven-year cycle. The *Neijing*, translated as *The Yellow Emperor's Classic of Medicine*, says that women are no longer able to conceive beyond a certain age. That age, forty-nine, is much different than Western statistics, which tag age thirty-five as the beginning of the end of women's fertility. Although forty-nine is probably out of the question for most women today, it does give women in their early forties hope, and certainly in my practice I've seen plenty of success in women around that age.

Kidney (Kid, for short) energy has a pilot light for the furnace of your life. It allows you to turn deep within to access your will and determination to feel the pulse of existence. To simplify, in Western medicine, Kid energy correlates to the adrenal glands, which sit atop the kidneys. Besides regulating metabolism and controlling blood pressure, the adrenal glands deliver the hormones our bodies need to respond appropriately when we are under stress, when we perceive danger, or when we experience high anxiety (the nervous system's fight-or-flight response). If we're under constant stress, our adrenals will keep churning out cortisol until they're exhausted or depleted. At that point, the pilot light has pretty much gone out and there's very little energy left for sex and certainly a much lower probability that conception will occur. It's as if the body is saying "now is not the time to make a baby." We see this in nature, as well. When a mammal feels threatened, she becomes fearful, her reproductive system shuts down, and she doesn't ovulate.

When the water element is out of balance and Kid energy is depleted, the predominant emotion is fear. The dream of having a child is the longing of the heart to experience love, to nurture, to create. When that can't happen, many women become afraid: *If I don't have a child by the age of forty, my life will be over.* For single women, fear is the energy they put forward as they look desperately for a mate or wonder if they can go it alone. And fear is what takes over when we live in the unknown. The antidotes for fear are compassion and forgiveness. Acknowledge the fear, sit with it. It can feel like it's lingering like a simmering flame on a stove whose burner has been left on. By wrapping our loving arms around our fears, we can acknowledge them, saying, "And this, too."

The fire element, or Heart energy, is the center of our mental and emotional states and, along with its other functions, governs the flow of blood throughout the body. Sometimes referred to as the "House of Spirit," this yin channel connects to the brain and the hypothalamus. If a woman experiences any trauma, chronic stress, or disruption in the flow of her life, the Heart energy responsible for opening the cervix for ovulation will close it down instead. In more anatomical terms, emotional stress directly affects the hypothalamus, which leads to pituitary dysfunction and delayed

ovulation. This happens quite frequently. Women under pressure to reproduce find that their cycles become irregular, which causes even more
stress because they can't predict when they will ovulate.

When the fire element is balanced, it helps us form healthy relationships
where we interact compassionately with others. Because of its connection
to Small Intestine energy, the fire element also helps us weigh our options
dispassionately and make sound decisions. According to traditional Chinese medicine's five-element theory, Small Intestine energy filters the
pure from the impure and decides what the Heart energy should focus
on physically, mentally, and emotionally. Like a minister to a king, Small
Intestine qi deals with incoming energies so that the Heart can center
on love and wisdom. When the fire element, or Heart energy, is depleted,
symptoms such as insomnia, heart palpitations, anxiety, and deep sadness
can result. The disappointment and defeat that couples feel when they
can't conceive further diminish their energy. It's hard to feel sexy when
the fire in the heart is low. Of course, if the fire is raging out of control, this
can also lead to an unbalanced state, fueling dissatisfaction and causing
an inability to commit or even compulsive sexual behavior, sometimes
labeled as sex addiction. The antidote is securing our place with love.

When the energies are balanced, the ancient Chinese say, Kidney essence
(our reproductive energy) rises upward, and Heart essence (love and passion) moves downward via the Chong meridian, and they join together.
Although the role of the Chong vessel (along with the other "extraordinary"
channels) in menstruation and fertility is discussed at length in chapter 11,
it's important to note here its role in establishing an intimate connection
between the heart and the uterus. Jeffrey Yuen, a Taoist monk and one of my
teachers, says the Chong meridian is the blueprint of life—it's what we pass
on to our offspring, so it needs to be balanced and our vital energy strength-
ened. If our children are to inherit that vitality, we want to conceive in love
and put off baby-making sex if we feel stressed, sick, or out of sorts.

How do you know if your Chong vessel is out of balance? Ask yourself the
following questions. If you answer yes to any of them, let your acupuncturist know; she can help clear this energy pathway.

Do you ever feel a sense of anxiety rushing up into your chest?

Do you also have cold hands and feet?

Have your menstrual cycles changed, producing less blood than before?

All the elements in traditional Chinese medicine contain a physical, mental, and emotional component and emphasize the point at which the body, mind, and spirit connect. The kidneys, for example, store jing, which corresponds to our primordial essence. This "essential qi," as jing is sometimes called, can be extended to the eggs and sperm, which contain the DNA essential for all life.

THE CRUCIAL IMPORTANCE OF ZHI

Traditional Chinese medicine believes that the spirit of the Kidney energy is zhi, which translates as the will to act or accomplish things and can manifest as the human desire to reproduce and thrive. The highest use of this zhi energy is to align with the Tao, the flow of the universe, in a state of nondoing or nonaction—*wuwei*, in Chinese. This doesn't mean that couples should stop having sex or should not do IUI or IVF. It simply means that our actions should be aligned with the natural order of the universe, in a state of effortless effort. The idea is to move forward without pushing back the river.

The zhi has a direct relationship with the shen of the heart, which is the spirit of the fire element. According to traditional Chinese medicine, shen is the center point of human awareness and our connection to the Divine. According to Lorie Dechar, author of *Five Spirits: Alchemical Acupuncture for Psychological and Spiritual Healing*, "The shen manifests in the radiance that shines from the eyes and a vibrant, flourishing quality of the complexion. . . . It is the fiery, yang spark of conscious awareness that is said to reside in the human heart. It is related to love and compassion."[2] We must strive to balance our energies—water and fire (yin and yang)—so we are able to connect love (Heart energy) with our innate desire to procreate (Kidney energy). When these two elements are healthy and in balance, the outpouring of love can manifest in conception.

It is love and compassion that nourish relationships, open us up to our intuitive nature, and help us know our true Self. When you truly know yourself, you can be authentic with your partner and communicate your heart's desires. Love can then blossom like a lotus flower, extending to the totality of who you are and ultimately connecting you with the oneness of the universe and the spirit of the unborn child. Love is that powerful. Call in love through your heart and move it down into your lower chakras, where it can unite with your reproductive energy to nurture and nourish your creative center.

To truly know yourself, you must let go of the fear and self-loathing that can surface when you feel that your body (and perhaps your relationship) have betrayed you. Yes, acupuncture and the right blend of herbs can support and nourish your body and begin to bring it back into stasis, and moxabustion, which is mugwort burned over acupuncture points, can really stoke the fire in your loins. But you must also commit to making lifestyle changes and renewing commitments that sustain you and bring you joy.

Mary's story is a wonderful example of the power of conscious choices and loving self-reflection. Mary, a patient of mine in West Hollywood, and her husband, Russ (pseudonyms to protect their privacy), wanted a child more than anything. By the time I met her, she had already been to a fertility doctor, suffered two miscarriages, and had two failed IVF transfers, in which none of her embryos were viable. Her conviction that their "failure" to conceive was all her fault prevented her from being able to make love with her husband. In fact, she could barely look at Russ without feeling shame and sadness.

When Mary and I began to talk, she told me that she worked long hours in a highly paid, very stressful executive position that she hated. She knew she should quit, but she couldn't. "I have to stay in my job," she said. "I get great insurance and we need that if we're going to have a baby." But the stress of her job and her lifestyle had already taken a toll. She ate only one meal a day (dinner), her menstrual cycle was irregular, and her hands and feet were always cold.

We began Mary's treatment by focusing on her eating habits, reestablishing a commitment to a healthy breakfast, lunch, and dinner, while slowly weaning her off her three-cups-a-day coffee fixation. In what TCM would call a clear sign of Chong meridian imbalance or blockage, soon after her two failed IVF treatments Mary reported acute anxiety that began in her belly and radiated up to her chest—a fitting metaphor for her belief that her body and her heart were broken. Acupuncture treatments helped rebalance her Chong meridian and contributed to healing not only her body, but her emotional state as well. Her symptoms improved even more when Mary made the brave decision to quit her job and take another one with more manageable hours and fewer responsibilities.

During all of this I gave Mary two homework assignments: keep a basal temperature chart so she could get to know her menstrual cycle and when she might be ovulating, and add a little red heart on the chart every day that she and her husband made love. The first time she brought in her chart I saw only one red heart. I gently reminded her that it's hard to make a baby naturally without making love. Mary confessed that she was afraid to make love because she was afraid of having another miscarriage. In Chinese medicine, Mary's fear, as well as the trauma she experienced during and after her two miscarriages, had caused her Heart and Kidney energies to shut down, which manifested as a low sex drive and anxiety. If a gate is closed, a person can be stuck in the dark. To help her, I needled the point on the Chong pathway called Kid 21, "Dark Gate," which Chinese medicine says will help her confront her fears by balancing her mind and her spirit. I then suggested herbs and nutritional supplements to strengthen her body and womb. Finally, I gave her and Russ exercises to do to help them regain their intimacy and the connection that they had lost along the way.

Mary credits my insistence that they make out as often as possible as what led to their eventually reconnecting with each other. She said they both were surprised at how deeply they felt each kiss—all the way down into their loins—and how quickly it drove them to make love with a renewed insistence and pleasure. Why? Chinese medicine says that Heart energy opens the tongue. Western medicine agrees but explains things a little differently. Research conducted in 2009 at Arizona State University shows that long, passionate kisses relieve stress and improve the body's ability to rest and relax by increasing parasympathetic nervous system activity and even lowering blood pressure and cholesterol. Sexy kisses also increase oxytocin (the "love hormone") to keep love alive—or reinvigorate it—and flood the body with plenty of dopamine to move couples on to the next level.[3]

Science writer Sheril Kirshenbaum, author of *The Science of Kissing: What the Lips Are Telling Us,* says that men prefer sloppy kisses because they can dose women with small amounts of libido-raising testosterone in their saliva. Over time, this can raise a woman's libido. Apparently that worked for Mary! Along with the acupuncture treatments and herbs I gave her to help heal her body, let go of fear, and open her heart, Mary says all that slow, passionate kissing certainly made sex fun and pleasurable again. A month later, she conceived their first child naturally—at age forty-two.

I saw Mary for treatments throughout her pregnancy, so we had an opportunity to talk more about what had happened that helped release her from her fears and her self-directed shame-and-blame game. She said she grew weary of always being afraid, of not taking chances because, in her mind anyway, she had already failed. As Ram Dass says, "Be love, embody love." It's so tempting to hold back and protect ourselves, to choose security over the unknown. But if we're not willing to open our hearts to one another, to our dreams, and be willing to fail, to hurt, to cry, then everything we desire will eventually be lost. There is no security, but there is always a return to love, to the energy of the heart, and to the home of the spirit.

Here are some of the exercises I gave Mary and her husband to help them reclaim the sacredness of their union, relight the flame in their hearts and the loins, and enjoy each other fully. Some of the exercises are taken from tantra yoga, an ancient body-based practice that connects divine force (Shakti, feminine energy) with pure consciousness (Shiva, masculine energy). Through this union, tantrikas say, we are connected to the whole of creation and to the Divine, with no beginning and no end.

Other exercises are taken from traditional Chinese medicine and Western sexual practices.

EXERCISE 1: KISSING

If it worked for Mary and Russ, chances are it will work for you, too. And it'll certainly be fun! Try making out like you did when you first discovered each other, with no goal in mind. Be fully present to your partner and simply engage in long, slow, passionate kisses.

EXERCISE 2: CONNECTING HEART-TO-HEART

Start by sitting in a comfortable cross-legged position facing your partner. If this position is uncomfortable, sit up on the edge of a folded blanket or yoga block (or simply find a position that works for both of you).

1. Begin by looking into each other's eyes. This can sometimes feel awkward or disagreeable, but see if you can stick with it for three to five minutes.
2. Place your left hand (receptive yin energy) flat in the middle of your partner's chest, at the heart center. Have your partner do the same to you—left hand in the middle of your chest. Hold your partner's right hand and continue to look into each other's eyes.
3. As you hold your right hands, begin to harmonize your breathing, inhaling and exhaling in unison. Don't try too hard or worry that you get off-sync. Just notice and breathe along with each other as much as possible. Stay with it for as long as you wish—three to five minutes, perhaps, working up to a full ten minutes. At the end, reach out to each other for a full-body embrace. Don't just hug at a physical level; embrace your partner with your whole being. As Dean Sluyter, author of *Natural Meditation*, puts it, "Hug their presence with your presence, their innocence with your innocence, their beingness with your beingness."[4]

EXERCISE 3: CONNECT WATER AND FIRE ENERGIES

Ask your partner to lie down on their stomach. Place one hand on their lower back, level with the second lumbar vertebra (which corresponds to Kidney energy), and one hand between their shoulder blades, around the fifth thoracic vertebra, behind the heart (which corresponds to Heart energy). Close your eyes and breathe all of your loving attention into your partner's body and heart. Then switch places.

EXERCISE 4: LAUGH OUT LOUD!

Patanjali, chronicler of the Yoga Sutras, the foundational treatise of yoga, says when you're suffering, cultivate the opposite. If you've been stressed, depressed, and anxious, flip the switch and be silly, watch dumb movies that make you laugh, and see the absurdity in some of the things you've been told to do on this baby-making journey. It may feel forced at first, but that's okay. You may also find it a welcome relief and a way to reset.

SEXUAL SECRET
Tasting the Love Nectar

The Taoists and tantrikas realized the importance of our secretions. According to these esoteric teachings, a woman produces three types of sexual secretions— one from her mouth, one from her breasts, and one from her yoni. Some say that orgasm changes the quality of saliva in our mouth and gives it healing properties when ingested. Try this: Right before you orgasm, (women) place your tongue on the roof of your mouth just behind the front teeth. After orgasm offer your tongue to your partner so they can suck the special saliva that is produced.

10

Setting the Stage

....

Remember the entrance to the sanctuary is inside you.

-RUMI

A COUPLE CAME TO SEE THE WISE CHINESE MASTER. They were unable to conceive and were sad and discouraged. He had a cure, he told them: Go get a couple of rabbits, a boy and a girl, put them in a cage in the bedroom and watch what happens. Within a few months the couple got pregnant. And while the wise master may not have known the old saying "You need to f**k like bunnies to make a baby," he was well aware of the power of suggestion, humor, and the effectiveness of feng shui, the ancient art of creating harmonious surroundings. While I don't advocate getting real bunnies, a pair of ceramic ones might serve as a lighthearted reminder of what the bedroom is for!

He had a point. Have you ever walked into a room and felt peaceful and calm? Or energized and inspired? Perhaps the colors were stimulating or the mood romantic. On the other hand, how turned-on do you feel upon entering a room where dirty clothes litter your unmade bed, the remnants of last night's snack and last week's cup of half-drunk coffee perched precariously on a stack of books and loose papers on your nightstand? How turned-on do you think it makes your partner feel?

It's important to create a sacred space for lovemaking, and even though we are going to spend some time talking about the bedroom, you can create a beautiful space in any room in your house.

THE BEDROOM

Tucked away from the center of the house, this special room is usually our sanctuary. It is the place in the house where we find refuge to recharge body and mind and to connect with our partner. Of course, to spice things up, hot sex can also happen in other places in the house, but the bedroom usually reigns supreme for comfort. So shut the door to keep all the good energy (qi) contained and to create a sensuous, loving atmosphere. Find that sweet spot of intimacy and relaxation using tools borrowed from feng shui, the ancient Chinese art of placing objects in such a way that a person can live in balance, good health, and harmony.

The term *feng shui* means "wind and water," two intersecting elements. Wind represents breath, energy, and the inner world, and water represents the physical, life-sustaining, outer world. By paying attention to our surroundings, we can maximize positive energy and minimize negative energy. If you've ever been in a house that has been feng-shuied, you probably noticed a sense of calm and ease, as though energy is flowing freely. Many of feng shui's concepts are practical ways to make living in our environment more enjoyable.

Clear the Clutter

Marie Kondo made quite a splash when she wrote *The Life-Changing Magic of Tidying Up*, in which she encouraged us all to sort through everything we own—books, photos, papers, clothing, even furniture. Touch it, hold it, and then decide whether to keep it or let it go. What particularly struck me was the author's insistence that we need to keep the stuff that "sparks joy."[1] I tell my patients that sorting and purging makes room for what we want to manifest in our lives that hasn't happened yet—and that includes babies.

Remove the Electronics

No cell phones, computers, tablets, or televisions in your bedroom, please. It's pretty common knowledge that such devices give off electromagnetic frequencies that can disturb sleep, but did you know that they can also distract from intimacy? My patient Gail complained that her husband sat in bed every night with his laptop, checking his email, barely even acknowledging her. That was bad enough, she said, but she had also heard that resting a computer on his lap could adversely affect his sperm. She wanted to know if that was true. I told her that an article published in the *Journal of Biomedical Physics and Engineering* noted that several studies showed that using laptop computers on the lap can adversely affect men's reproductive health. The article stated that the heat from a laptop computer warms a man's scrotum, while "the electromagnetic fields generated by [the] laptop's internal electronic circuits, as well as the Wi-Fi radio frequency radiation hazards (in a Wi-Fi connected laptop), may decrease sperm quality."[2] And if that isn't bad enough, the artificial light these electronics give off can disrupt circadian rhythms, which messes with sleep patterns—and disrupted sleep can negatively affect fertility, according to a 2015 study published in *Cell Reports*.[3] Same thing goes for cell phones, apparently: wearing phones on your person and talking on them may negatively affect sperm quality. For Gail, her bedroom had become a workroom. Once she suggested to her husband that they remove all electronics from the bedroom, their sex life returned. And if you have a TV in the bedroom, just cover it with a cloth when you're not using it, or better yet, put it in a cabinet.

Choose Your Colors

Most feng shui experts say stick with natural earth tones in the bedroom, such as beige or cream, or warming colors such as peach or pink. To add a little pizzazz, you can accent with different shades of red—the color of the fire element—which will increase yang energy. Pillows of crimson or pomegranate, for example, are known to have activating qualities. Of course, if there's already a lot of stimulating energy in the room, red might be too much. In her book *Feng Shui Your Life*, Jayme Barrett says to cool things down, "go with light greens, blues, and lavender. Blue calms; pinks and peaches invite love and romance."[4]

Keep the Decor Neutral

This goes for fabrics as well. It's best to choose soft materials, organic if possible. It's always nice to have materials like silk and cotton against your skin; I even encourage couples to invest in a silk-and-cotton pillow for the woman to place under her tush after sex to help keep the sperm in. I bought a beautiful Indian pillow, but its raised gold threads made it too scratchy to use on my bed, so I relegated it to my chair instead. Obviously, comfort is key.

Think about Your Bed

Might be time to invest in a new mattress, one that's not too soft, not too hard, and above all, comfortable—and if you can afford it, organic. The best position for your bed, feng shui experts say, is the back corner against the wall (for stability), with your head pointing east. If that's not possible, don't worry. Try to arrange the bed so it's not directly facing a door, underneath a beam, or under a window. Also, to ensure a balanced relationship, make sure you can get in and out of the bed on both sides. Jayme Barrett also adds that your bed should be "in a spot you can't wait to jump into."[5] One final furniture caveat: beware of sharp, pointy corners, which feng shui folks call "poison arrows." Soften those edges with pillows or throw blankets— anything that will distract your attention away from the sharp corners.

Cover the Mirrors

Sure, we all know about mirrors on the ceiling and how watching yourself making love can be a fun way to spice up your sex life. But the problem with this is that you end up focusing *outside*, on the image of yourself making love, and neglect being fully engaged with your partner. Also, this might not be great if you have a negative body image. Instead, I recommend practicing the mirror exercise in the Five-Element Lover's Wheel in chapter 8. Besides, if you're following traditional feng shui principles, mirrors don't belong in the bedroom—they're too stimulating and they tend to multiply what they see. If you do have mirrors, covering them at night will help ensure a peaceful sleep after the activities of the evening.

Dim the Lights

I must say I'm a big fan of mood lighting in the bedroom. I like to be able to look into my partner's eyes when we make love, and dim lighting works. If you don't have dimmer switches, you can place a beautiful silk scarf, preferably in red, over a bedside lamp, light a few nontoxic candles, or try a Himalayan salt-crystal lamp. The warm glow these lamps give off is reminiscent of a golden sunset, and I always feel they can turn any room into a haven of sensual delight. They even purportedly have a few health benefits: some practitioners say they contribute to cleansing and deodor- izing the air, neutralizing electromagnetic radiation, and improving sleep and mood. And don't place a ceiling light directly over your bed—it's con- sidered inauspicious and maybe even bad for your liver and your eyesight, according to feng shui.

Enhance Air Quality

I live in Los Angeles, not exactly known for its stellar air quality. When Alex and I were trying to get pregnant I invested in a very expensive HEPA filter, which I turned on at night—Alex used to refer to it as "the jet engine." But I know he was glad we had one since research has suggested that dirty air may adversely affect sperm parameters. As well, dust often and air out the room by opening the windows.

Outfit the Relationship Corner

The rear right side of the bedroom is considered the relationship corner. How's yours looking? Might be time to give it a little attention. Choose symbols of love for the two of you—perhaps your wedding picture or a beautiful piece of art, which represents the power of your commitment. I'm a big fan of erotic sculpture—they make me think of Auguste Rodin's *The Kiss* and his love affair with sculptor Camille Claudel. Place a small vase of fresh flowers in shades of pink and red, along with a couple of beeswax or coconut wax candles on a table in this corner. Make sure the candles have nontoxic wicks and are scented with 100 percent natural essential oils. Lighting the candles gives a pretty clear signal that your special togetherness time is about to begin. Keep photographs of parents, children, and friends out of the bedroom—the focus should be on partner-ship. I don't really encourage pets in the bedroom while you're trying to conceive either—I feel like they're too distracting (this goes for aquariums, too). Feng shui says they're too stimulating.

ALTARS

I once was invited into a cottage in the small town of Cusco, in the foot-hills of Peru, on my way to hike the Inca trail to Machu Picchu. The first thing I noticed were guinea pigs eating greens on the dirt floor—it turns out they're quite a delicacy in Peru. I then saw two twin beds with metal headboards on my left; on the right stood a black stone fireplace with a shelf built into a stone wall. The three skulls perched there—part of the family's altar—seemed to stare right at me even though there were no eyes in the hollow sockets. The tour guide began to tell us the meaning of all the items on the shelf. The skulls represented the blessings of their ances-tors, he said, and an Incan cross was revered for its spiritual presence. As he explained the significance of the other items—animal carvings, a special candle, and a selection of fresh yellow flowers—my eyes fixated on the big-gest figure up there that he had somehow failed to mention: an eight-inch black stone penis. So of course I had to ask: what's the meaning of *that*?

He blushed, and before he could reply I blurted, "Does it have to do with fertility?" Relieved he didn't have to answer my question, he quickly shook his head yes. At Machu Picchu, I caught a glimpse of what looked like another penis stone, complete with testicles, imbedded in the rocks on a wall. I turned to my fourteen-year-old son and asked, "Is that what I think it is?" "Yup," he said, "that's a penis and two balls alright." Obviously, fertility was prized by the Incas. On the way home I purchased a stone phallus to place on my own altar to represent creation.

In many cultures, an altar—often set on a platform or table—is a center for worship. In the Judeo-Christian tradition, altars represent the place where the Divine and human worlds interact. Although altars for sacri-ficial offerings can be found in many churches, what I'm talking about here are personal altars. For example, in Chinese culture, altars and shrines are everywhere, even in the back corner of restaurants, and they're often infused with incense. In Bali, daily offerings of beautiful flowers, incense, and other items are put in woven baskets and placed on home altars as well as in Balinese temples to appease the various gods and demons of Balinese Hinduism. In Japanese restaurants you'll frequently see statues of lucky cats displayed on shelves. These lucky cats come in a variety of colors and symbolize different things. For example, the tri-color cat is good for luck, wealth, and prosperity, while pink cats are said to be good for love, relationships, and romance. Hindus believe that an altar for worship of the Divine is most powerful when it's placed in the northeast corner of a room. The altar may include incense, a lamp, bells, and offerings of fresh flowers; at its center almost always is a statue of a spiritual deity called a *murti*, a sacred image that embodies a god or goddess.

An altar in your home can be a place for meditation or a place of beauty, where you invoke the sacred with various symbols of importance to you. For women who want to conceive, creating an altar with special items of significance is a great way to put attention on the sacred and usher in intimacy, love, and fertility. Designing an altar together allows the two of you to create something powerful that you both can relate to. Here are a few suggestions to make that happen:

1. Find a place in your home for the altar and take some time organizing the physical space so that it's free of clutter and chaos. The altar can go anywhere that feels special to you: in your bedroom, a corner of your living room, meditation room, or even a little nook off the kitchen. If you wish, use some sage to purify or sanctify the space. Simply light a piece, blow out the flame, and let it smolder (like incense). Using your hands, you can direct some of the smoke, bringing it up to your face and down your body, like you're giving yourself a smoke bath. Then wave the smoke slowly around the space you have chosen to place your altar. When you're finished, place the sage in a clay bowl or an abalone shell. This practice is known as smudging. I prefer palo santo, "holy wood," which grows on the coast of South America, said to keep

away not only mosquitoes but also bad vibes. It's not as smoky as sage and I love the smell of it. I burn it on my altar as incense.

2. Choose a beautiful piece of fabric made of natural materials for your altar cloth, on which you can place items that have spiritual significance or a special connection for the two of you. Before laying down the items you've chosen, take a few moments to call forth abundance, fertility, and love. Anything else you'd like to visualize together, do that now.

3. Choose your items. Be creative, adding stones, bells, seeds—anything that symbolizes fertility or represents your journey together. They need not be religious or ancient, just infused with special meaning. My friend Lisa has several altars she's created. One she particularly loves has several dolphins on it. For her, these figurines serve as a reminder to breathe. She says, "Navigating the deep waters of your emotions? Breathe. Feeling overwhelmed? Breathe." You get the idea. Below I've listed a few items that represent fertility. No doubt you'll come up with others that have meaning for you.

Shiva Lingam Stone

These egg-shaped stones made of cryptocrystalline quartz are found on the sacred Narmada River, in Onkar Mandhata, India. They come in all different sizes, ranging from ones that fit in the palm of your hand to enormous ones up to eleven feet long. The egg shape depicts the male reproductive organ (the lingam) of Lord Shiva, and some say the special markings on the stone represent female energy—an obvious metaphor for fertility and creation. Place one on your altar to bring in the energy of conception; use it during meditation by placing it in palm of your hand.

Lotus Flower

This beautiful flower blossoms out of muddy waters and in Eastern tradition symbolizes our ability to rise above difficult circumstances. This certainly can apply to the challenges we face when we're trying to conceive. A painting or photograph placed on your altar will remind you that joy, life, and light can spring from despair and darkness.

Bells

Bells in the form of wind chimes call good energy into a home, according to feng shui experts. In Hinduism the bell is a fertility symbol—the outside is shaped like a vulva and the inside contains the gong, signifying the penis.

Pomegranate

Feng shui says that the seeds of a pomegranate symbolize fertility. Like an ovary, the pomegranate has many seeds and therefore great life potential. Buy small red marbles and place them in a bowl on your altar to symbolize pomegranate seeds.

Dragons

In Eastern traditions, dragons symbolize sexuality, wisdom, fertility, and longevity, as well as abundance and good fortune. Place one on your bedroom altar if you need more yang energy—in other words, if you need to ignite the sexual fire in yourself or your partner.

Elephants

In feng shui it is a common practice to place a pair of elephants in the bedroom to activate the energy of conception. In the Hindu tradition, Ganesha (Ganapati), a cute, potbellied deity resembling an elephant, is said to remove obstacles. Use him on your altar to overcome hurdles in the fertility process.

Gems and Crystals

The Chinese, Indians, Greeks, Mayans, Tibetans, and other traditional cultures have used stones, rocks, and crystals for healing. Sensual to the touch and lovely to gaze at, crystals and stones are wonderful adornments to place on your altar and also to wear. Heather Askinosie, co-founder of Energy Muse, a blog and crystal shop, and the co-author of *Crystal Muse*, says when she was going through her fertility journey she used stones like carnelian, turquoise, and citrine to heal and balance her second and third chakras. "The whole energy of the earth is a tool for healing," she says.[6]

Choose the stones and crystals that resonate most for you. Here are a few that are known to promote fertility and enliven sexuality:

MOONSTONE: Connected to the energies of the moon, wear moonstone when you want to regulate your menstrual cycle or boost fertility; it is also known to be calming.

ROSE QUARTZ: The stone of love, rose quartz can help with sexual difficulties and is one of the main stones used to increase fertility. Wear it as a bracelet or put it on your altar.

RED CARNELIAN: The color of this form of carnelian, a mixture of red and orange, represents passion and the fire element. It stimulates the sacral and second chakras and increases sensuality.

RED JASPER: Used to promote strength and endurance, clear the mind, and invigorate the libido, red jasper is a stone of passion and protection, and it increases sexual stamina.

SHUNGITE: A two-billion-year-old ancient healing stone, shungite is found only in Karelia, Russia. According to Heather Askinosie, the elite shungite—the rarest type because it contains the most carbon—is known as the "stone of fruition" because "it brings forth positive blessings and positive results."[7] She says it relieves stress, anxiety, and insomnia and boosts overall energy.

Paintings and Photographs

Photographs or paintings can include your ancestors, mentors, spiritual teachers, friends, loved ones who have passed, or any other inspirational people you would like to honor.

Fertility Figures

African female fertility figures known as Akua Ba, made of wood, beads, and string, are traditionally "used in a variety of contexts; primarily, however, they are consecrated by priests and carried by women who hope to conceive a child."[8] According to legend, when a woman named Akua couldn't conceive a child, she conferred with a priest, who told her to carry such a statue strapped to her back. It worked—she gave birth to a baby girl. I bought one when I found out that my husband and I were carriers of Tay-Sachs, a genetic disorder, and we weren't sure if the child I was carrying was okay. I placed this statue on my altar to remind me to have faith in the unknown, like Akua did.

Goddesses

Many traditions pay homage to the Divine Feminine by honoring the Goddess in her many forms. Sometimes we see her with a spiral on her belly representing a circle moving forward in time. Celtic people used a triple spiral O to represent the Goddess. Some of my favorites forms of the Divine Feminine include:

APHRODITE, the Greek goddess of passion and love. She helps women connect with their primal sexuality and helps both genders get in touch with their intuitive feminine nature, feel proud of their bodies, and be receptive. Use her when you want to call forth more sensuality.

KUAN YIN, the goddess of compassion and mercy, the gentle mother. Call on her when you want to bring compassion to yourself and others and connect to the love in your heart. *Om Mani Padme Hum*—this Buddhist mantra is often used to call forth Kuan Yin.

LAKSHMI, the Hindu goddess of prosperity, beauty, power, and fertility. She is the consort of Lord Vishnu and is often displayed at Hindu weddings. Call on her when you need reassurance that everything will work out.

MUSIC

"And in the end, the love you take is equal to the love you make." Every time I hear "The End," from the Beatles' *Abbey Road*, I feel the power of love and connection, and tears well up in my eyes. When I listen to Led Zeppelin's "Stairway to Heaven," it takes me back to my first kiss—I can actually feel the sensation of that kiss in my body. Music engages our emotions and memories because it is processed in the areas of the brain that control memories, both implicit (amygdala) and explicit (hippocampus). According to various studies, these parts of the brain decode associated emotions and context with music, which is why I associate "Stairway to Heaven" with something that happened many years ago. Listening to music you love releases dopamine, the "love-at-first-sight" chemical, in the reward center of the brain.

Sounds and music especially help open the psyche and clear the mind and heart as they prepare the body for lovemaking. When you light some candles and put on your favorite tunes, you are creating an atmosphere of sensuality and literally setting the stage. Can you see why music would be such a lovely addition to your intimacy tool kit? And don't forget that nature also has lovely sounds such as birdcalls, ocean waves, crickets, or tree frogs. Making love in nature can be delightful for the senses. When you can't make it outside you can always bring the outdoors into your bedroom via nature recordings.

Paying attention to your environment by making your bedroom a pleasure zone, choosing decor that brings in passion, creating a special altar, and using music are all ways to set the stage for heightened lovemaking. There are no rules, only your own creativity and inspiration. Grace your life with the realization that the beauty inside you and your partner can be reflected on the outside, in your surroundings. If all this seems too overwhelming, start with a single change. After all, Confucius says, "The man who moves a mountain begins by carrying away small stones."

SEXUAL SECRET
Don't Vacuum under the Bed

To up your fertility quotient, Chinese folklore says to place a cup of uncooked rice under the bed, in the center. I asked Rodika Tchi, a private feng shui consultant whose company, Tchi Consulting, is based in Vancouver, BC, to explain that tradition. She said that rice is a Chinese symbol of fertility and abundance, which "mostly works because of the strong cultural belief in it. So, honestly, you can use any other symbol that has meaning for you," she says. "As long as you have faith in it, it will work as well as a bowl of rice." But feng shui says don't store anything—and don't even dust—under your bed until your child is born, so you don't disturb the energy of fertility. "The reason for not vacuuming under the bed is to create a strong (and undisturbed) energetic grounding," she says. "Basically, it's to have a very settled, safe, and supportive energy to help conception."

11

Healing Trauma,
Letting Go of Shame

....

When we say a simple and sincere yes to life,
yes to death, yes to the ego's own dissolving,
we don't have to struggle anymore.
It becomes a new way of navigating through life.
Flow is what navigates us through life—not concepts,
not ideas, not what we should or shouldn't do,
not what's right or wrong.

—ADYASHANTI

I AM A HUGE FAN OF OPRAH. She has done what she encourages all of us to do: "Turn your wounds into wisdom." She knows what it's like to suffer sexual abuse and heal from it. And while she didn't go on to have children, she did put her creative energy to good use, to stimulate, educate, entertain, motivate, and inspire us all. She believes that whatever our wounds are, wherever our traumas emerge from, we can grow from them, heal, and go on to make a difference in the world. If you have had your own traumas, use this chapter for suggestions to get back to pleasure and love, and from that place create intimacy that has no choice but to bring life forward.

For those of you who suffer from sexual trauma, please know you're not alone. In my many years of treating women and men for sexual dysfunction and infertility challenges, I've seen hundreds of ways that trauma has played a role in their distress: ambivalence or aversion to touch or sexual penetration, to their own bodies, and even to the idea of parenthood—all of which spill over into their day-to-day relationships and, in some cases, prevent them from achieving their goals.

Before we dive too far into how trauma can adversely affect your ability to conceive, let's take a moment to define it. Trauma is a person's reaction to an event that overwhelms his or her ability to cope or integrate it. Trauma for women and men can stem from unprocessed emotions—wounds from childhood, adolescence, or young adulthood caused by physical, emotional, or sexual abuse; negative messages about sexuality; betrayal, self-loathing, addiction, and dishonesty; old memories that surface from having an abortion or a string of miscarriages. And finally, trauma can emerge from the stress of trying to conceive in the first place, made even worse for couples who must choose medically assisted fertility treatments. Trauma shows up as negative thoughts and self-criticism; as anxiety, fear, and sadness in the emotional body, which can't be expressed or released; and in the somatic body as physical conditions—vulvar pain in women, for example, and erection or ejaculating difficulties in men. All of these forms of trauma can keep women and men from experiencing sexual pleasure.

Trauma is highly personal—no two people react to difficult experiences in the same way. For example, Ava, a patient of mine, discovered many years ago that she had gotten genital herpes from a boyfriend who lied to her throughout their relationship. Now, many women and men I've worked with have confessed to having herpes, too—after all, it's a pretty common condition. And many of these folks have been able to accept it as an unfortunate reminder of their not-so-skillful past. Not Ava. She felt such unrelenting shame around her diagnosis that it deeply affected her ability to have a loving relationship with a man—for more than twenty years. When she got married, she insisted her husband wear a condom whenever they made love. When they were ready to have a child, she let him cut a hole in the tip of it.

Neuroscientists believe that trauma resides in the amygdala, the part of the limbic system where emotions are stored, but not language or speech. Hazel Williams-Carter, a traumacologist, healer, and founder of healingtraumacenter.com, explains that the amygdala is home of implicit, or emotional, memory. This part of the brain uses past experiences in the form of emotions and sensations to remember things without actually thinking about them. The amygdala responds not only to real fears (or other emotions), but also to the *memory* of fear. "For this reason, people who have been traumatized may live with implicit memories of the terror, anger, and sadness generated by the trauma," she says. This surfaced recently for Angela, a patient of mine who admitted that she hated having her breasts touched because she had been molested by her father. Whenever her partner goes to touch her breasts, she recoils; she wants to feel turned-on, but her amygdala registers fear and rage. She and her partner are working on ways to be intimate without triggering old, unprocessed emotions. Communication, as always, is key.

Trauma isn't necessarily tied to the past for couples trying hard to conceive. The fertility journey itself can be fraught with so many disappointments and conflicted feelings to work through, all of which takes a toll on a couple's ability to stay positive and connected. Women frequently complain to me that they get retraumatized every time their doctor reminds them that their eggs are "old," or tells them they have a slim-to-none chance of ever conceiving. They feel inadequate, ashamed, and depressed, which in turn affects their ability to be present in their intimate relationship and in their relationship with friends and co-workers. They end up blaming their partners and shunning their friends.

Working through trauma requires help. Forgiveness work, acupuncture, ritual, trauma-sensitive yoga, spiritual guidance—these are all tools that can help release stuck emotions. They all involve the body, not just the mind, because, as trauma experts will tell you, trauma lives in the body and needs to be released from the body. Talk therapy alone doesn't work because recounting your story can retrigger your nervous system and send you right back into fight-flight-freeze mode, as though the event were happening all over again.

ACUPUNCTURE AND THE EIGHT EXTRAORDINARY VESSELS

Much of my understanding of trauma and Chinese medicine comes from my teacher Jeffrey Yuen, an eighty-eighth generation Taoist priest of the Jade Purity School, Lao Tzu sect, and a twenty-sixth generation priest of the Complete Reality School, Dragon Gate sect—and a highly sought-after teacher of traditional Chinese medicine. As it turns out, acupuncture and TCM have a lot to offer anyone suffering from trauma, whether that trauma originates from an accident, the death of a loved one, childhood sexual abuse, or sexual dysfunction. Problems exist, the masters say, when we get separated from our authentic self and we don't do the work to understand what we've inherited physically and emotionally. The goal of TCM is to bring you to back to your authentic self, your true essence, which is never wounded or traumatized. Your authentic self, as Lonny Jarrett, author of *The Clinical Practice of Chinese Medicine*, explains, "is fully formed, always complete, and desires nothing except to be expressed."[1]

To express our authentic self, Chinese medicine calls on the Eight Extraordinary Vessels (a.k.a., the Eight Extra Channels), the pathways of energy that supply all the meridians of the body with life force and blood. In an article she wrote for *Acupuncture Today*, Mary Elizabeth Wakefield, LAc, Dipl.Ac., MS, says that the Chinese term for these eight vessels, Qi Jing Ba Mai, describes them best. She explains: "Qi is the energy that is likened to an 'ah-ha'—a flash of enlightened understanding. Jing penetrates our ancestral roots and makes up our DNA matrix—it is the precious essence of life. Ba means 'eight.' Mai symbolizes the movement in the meridians."

Much like the chakras in yoga, which are also powerful energy centers, the Qi Jing Ba Mai can become blocked by unresolved emotions or traumatic experiences. To heal trauma, we must address our wounds and release the stuck energy from these pathways. It's vital that we do this so that we don't accidentally pass these patterns on to the next generation.

Working with the Eight Extraordinary Vessels is TCM's way of reversing epigenetic inheritance. Epigenetic inheritance, according to Bruce Lipton, PhD, a stem-cell biologist and author of *The Biology of Belief*, is the understanding that "all the cells of your body are affected by your thoughts."[2] Beyond that, epigenetic researchers have found that those cells are also affected by the trauma we inherit from our parents and grandparents. This inheritance can alter gene activity without disturbing our DNA. The good news is that we can begin to reverse such epigenetic changes. In other words, we can release stuck emotions from our own experiences as well as those we've inherited, and this can stop us from passing them down to our own children. One way to do this is through the eight extra channels.

Eight Extraordinary Vessels work is pretty complex, so I don't want to give you the impression that I'm offering a one-size-fits-all healing. There's no such thing. I'm merely presenting a basic understanding of what these channels are and what they mean, along with some suggestions that may resonate with you. If you want to dive deeper, I invite you to find an acupuncturist who is familiar with these vessels.

Chong Mai: Penetrating Vessel

The Chong Mai invites us to understand ourselves and how we have arrived at where we are. Home of our ancestral inheritance, it is what we pass along to our offspring. And yes, that includes our own traumas as well as those of our parents, grandparents, and on and on down the ancestral line. The reproductive organs are part of this vessel, too. Some say that energetically the uterus holds on to and stores these unprocessed emotions, until they can be seen, acknowledged, and released. So it's easy to see how trauma can be transferred to our children before they even come into the world. Stories of not being wanted—like the mother who told her daughter, "Don't have kids, they are such a big burden," are held in this vessel and can destabilize it. So can anxiety, especially if your parents and or grandparents suffered from it. Being a victim of sexual violence can cause the Chong Mai and the Ren Mai to shut down.

When Chong Mai is balanced (mentioned in chapter 8 as well), our reproductive energy (Kidney essence) rises up toward the heart as the Heart essence (love and passion) moves downward. The Chong Mai is the pathway they travel to join together. That pathway should be clear of obstacles (traumas, sorrows, unprocessed emotions) so that our children can inherit vitality, strength, and a loving heart. To ensure that, we want to conceive in love, not when we're full of anxiety, distrust, and confusion.

Ren Mai: Conception Vessel

The name says it all: this meridian nourishes life. What seeds do we want to plant, nurture, and give birth to? The Ren Mai, which regulates reproductive function, controls all aspects of a woman's natural cycle—conception, fertility, pregnancy, puberty, and menopause. Furthermore, this vessel asks *Who am I? How was I nurtured by a primary caretaker? Did I get enough care?*

Ren Mai trauma can happen as a result of childhood neglect or abuse. Perhaps as a child you had primary caretakers who weren't attentive, who didn't help you learn to emotionally self-regulate, or were abusive. All of these memories leave a residue in the Ren Mai that can affect your ability to be intimate, feel worthy of love, or capacity for comforting yourself. These insecurities and traumas can manifest as an excessive need to be validated, needed, or loved by others, as well as a tendency to overeat or overindulge in drugs, alcohol, or inappropriate sexual behavior. The Ren Mai can also become unbalanced if your primary caretaker in childhood was overprotective and prevented you from exploring on your own. As an adult, this imbalance, seen as stagnation of qi in the abdomen, can lead to anxiety and insecurity.

To balance Ren Mai, the focus becomes "How can I love myself more?" Self-care is the first step to true healing. It may take a combination of talk therapy, loving-kindness meditation, acupuncture, and body-based practices like yoga and qigong to begin to feel more deserving of love and to learn how to honor yourself. The late Ray Rubio, founder of the American Board of Oriental Reproductive Medicine, once said, "We can't let the past define us. We must know our story, share our story and know how to do rewrites."[3] That's not always as easy or comfortable as it sounds, of course. But, Brené Brown, PhD, a research professor at the University of Houston, Texas, and a prolific author who talks and writes about vulnerability and shame, says, "Owning our story can be hard but not nearly as difficult as spending our lives running from it. . . . Only when we are brave enough to explore the darkness will we discover the infinite power of our light."[4]

CHONG AND REN MAI DYSFUNCTION: DIANE'S STORY

When Diane's mother, Azim, was sick from uterine cancer, Diane asked her if she had had to endure female genital mutilation as a child growing up in Egypt. Azim nodded her head. She revealed that her father died when she was five years old and that she and her sister went to live with their aunts. The aunts decided that the girls' pleasure center should be taken away so that they would "be obedient," insuring, Diane figured, that they would never be interested in men or leave the home. Azim eventually married and gave birth to two children. But she never went to see a gynecologist for a pap smear or an evaluation, even after she began bleeding at age sixty-four. Azim died of cancer not long after that conversation, and now Diane was in my office, hoping that acupuncture could stop her own uterine bleeding caused by a large fibroid that had appeared during her mother's illness. After Diane shared her story, I offered a possible solution. I told her that in Chinese medicine the uterus is called an "extraordinary" organ for several reasons: it is a vessel that holds a child; it discharges menstrual blood; and many say it energetically holds on to emotions lodged there, making it more difficult for them to be released. Perhaps Diane's job now—beyond grieving her mother's passing—was to heal the trauma she had inherited. This trauma was stored in her Chong Mai and Ren Mai vessels; she needed to release it so she could untie the binds that kept her life so deeply entwined with the suffering of her mother. Only then could she heal and bring more pleasure into her own life. Diane began her journey with me and her bleeding from the fibroid stopped. In fact, her menstrual cycles returned to normal and she began to date. Knowing that she would want children of her own someday, I encouraged Diane to get checked out by her ob-gyn.

Du Mai: Governing Vessel

Beginning at the perineum and moving up the spine, the Du Mai joins the Ren and Chong vessels in the *Who am I?* inquiry. The Du Mai, also called the Vessel of Individuality, is the body's yang aspect and presides over our individuation, the process of becoming self-aware or self-actualized. It's evident in children as they go from crawling to walking and begin to explore a world that includes more than just their primary caregiver. Adolescence is the second phase of individuation, when a young person discovers a sense of self distinct from, and not dependent on, the approval of their parents or caregivers. When there is weakness in this vessel, adults lack the motivation to go forward and often, instead of persevering, will give up, retreat, or slip into depression. Some describe feeling as though their strength has run out and, in terms of baby-making, they say trying to conceive is "just too much work." In the face of loss or disappointment such as a miscarriage or failed IVFs, they may be too scared to try again. On the other hand, a person with a Du Mai excess has a pretty rigid way of looking at the world and can get stuck in a "my way or the highway" mentality.

To balance this vessel it's important to reflect on what motivates you. What keeps you from moving forward with your dreams and desires? What are you afraid of? If a deficient or excessive Du Mai is preventing you from having a loving relationship, you may want to get help from a life coach, sexologist, or fertility specialist; an acupuncturist can suggest treatments and herbs to increase your motivation and even your sex drive. Practice yoga or qigong to gain flexibility—a flexible body can yield a flexible mind.

In life, we need a good balance of Ren Mai and Du Mai energies; in other words, a healthy sense of who we are, knowledge of where we want to go, and the ability to make it happen. Jeffrey Yuen says that we get the resources we need to create our destiny from these three vessels: the Chong gives us our blueprint, the Ren supplies the lumber, and the Du Mai provides construction.

Yin Wei Mai and Yang Wei Mai (Linking Vessels)

The two Wei vessels are like ropes or nets that hold things in place both structurally and psychologically, and they have to do with the aging process. They ask the question *What is my life's purpose?* When the Wei vessels do their job, we can meet life's challenges with more equanimity and grace and can bounce back from adversity. A strong Yang Wei vessel protects us from disease and external negativity, while Yin Wei nourishes us from the inside. When our Yang Wei is stable enough to withstand outside turmoil, we know how to choose actions that support us. Reaching out to those we know we can rely on—family, friends, mentors—can shore up the Yang Wei. So can being part of a community—perhaps joining a meditation circle or a church or support group. When our Yin Wei is strong, we know how to find what we need to feel more resilient, to be able to meet and withstand our internal turmoil and confusion. Conversely, a loose Yin Wei "net" can manifest physically as pain in the chest or around the heart. Emotionally, we may have trouble divorcing ourselves from past disappointments; we get caught in the past, stuck in the "if onlys," losing sight of where we're going.

To balance or strengthen the Yin Wei, it's important to acknowledge your feelings—all of them, without judgment. When you feel scared or ashamed, for example, instead of denying that you feel this way, you must commit to sitting with the fear and shame. In doing so, you may realize that the emotion is attached to the past and is trying to keep you there, too. Or you may discover that it isn't yours to begin with. If you have a tendency to complain about everything, once you sit with it you may realize that your mother used to complain all the time, too. You can then tell yourself that you have the power to feel those feelings, but you also have the power to release them—with gratitude. This unhooks the place in yourself where the energy in the net is bound up. As you take a look within, see if you can discover the places that feel stuck or constricted—perhaps the throat, your chest, or your pelvis. Chances are that's where you hold on to feelings you'd rather not look at. Breathe there—slow, easy, and steady breaths. Offer loving-kindness to the feelings you've harbored for so long and gratitude for their willingness to let go of you.

Yin Qiao Mei and Yang Qiao Mei (Vessels of One's Stance)

These pathways originate in the ankles and go to the eyes. How we stand in the present-day awareness of who we are is predicated on what our childhood experiences were. We can take our place in society when we know who we are.

Yin Qiao asks the questions *Am I comfortable in my body? Do I know who I am, even in the darkest aspects of myself?* When Yin Qiao is not in balance, all you want to do to is close out the world so no one can see how broken you feel. This is common in patients who are struggling with conceiving. They don't want to go to baby showers and they dread dinners with friends who have given birth already or who can't wait to share the news of their own pregnancies. They want to keep their distance from anything that could remind them of their "failure." I certainly am not interested in judging *that* inclination. What I am interested in is helping them strengthen their Yin Qiao Mei, which can address their feelings of inadequacy, their fear that they are not whole because they haven't conceived yet. One way to do that is by working with an acupuncturist. But Yin Qiao also invites us to practice loving-kindness and self-love *in the moment.* A powerful reminder comes from Theravada Buddhist teacher Ajahn Sumedho, who says, "Right now, it's like this"—a great mantra to help us stay in the present, with compassionate attention.

The Yang Qiao asks the questions *How do I move in the external world? Do I have a sense of ease in my body? Can I stand straight and tall?* Chronic pain in the neck, shoulders, and hips generally indicates imbalance in the Yang Qiao. This happens when you are moving forward at lightning speed, going from one thing to another, focusing on a single goal at the expense of everything else. It's when you don't know when or how to stop. To bring the Yang Qiao back into balance it's best to close your eyes and go inward toward the Yin Qiao. In other words: Stop. Listen. Feel. I encourage couples who have been using fertility drugs month after month without results to consider taking a break for a bit. Allow the nervous and immune systems to reregulate, and give the mind a chance to quiet down.

Dai Mei: Belt Vessel

Wrapped snugly around our lower area like a belt, this vessel guides and supports the qi of the uterus and that of the many energy pathways that flow through the torso. It is also where our body stores any trauma we've experienced from being violated and any deeply held sentiments we can't allow ourselves to feel. Sometimes people gain weight around their middle as a way of protecting themselves from unwanted advances or for other emotional reasons. Others may experience lower back pain that wraps around to the front. These are Dai Mei imbalances; others may present as fibroids, cysts, painful periods, painful intercourse, or prostatitis. A weakened vessel can even lead to miscarriage or uterine prolapse. The classic Chinese medicine texts say that an excess of Dai Mei can feel as though you're carrying five thousand coins on your back. So the question becomes *What are you carrying that no longer serves you?*

When the Dai Mei energy is stuck and the qi is not moving, I recommend using a rebozo, a very long, woven scarf used by Mesoamerican indigenous peoples. Midwives and doulas use these scarves to aid in labor and birthing. I find them helpful to get the uterine and pelvic qi unstuck or to strengthen a weakened Dai Mei, which can happen after a miscarriage. To move stuck qi, lie on your back and position the rebozo underneath your hips. Have your partner or a friend hold on to the ends of the rebozo and gently shake it back and forth, vigorously enough that you feel some shimmying in your hips. If your Dai meridian needs tightening because of the trauma of miscarriage, ask your partner to wrap the scarf around your womb center and tighten it like a belt.

METHODS OF HEALING TRAUMA

As I said, there are many ways to address the unprocessed feelings that we harbor and that prevent us from being in a loving and fertile relationship—with ourselves and with others. You may find one or more of the following to be particularly useful.

continues

Trauma-Sensitive Yoga

If you suffer from sexual trauma or other unprocessed emotions, finding a trauma-sensitive yoga class (or hiring a trauma-sensitive yoga teacher for private sessions) can be quite beneficial. David Emerson, author of *Overcoming Trauma through Yoga*, told me he believes survivors need to learn how to take their power back. But, he says, "Empowerment can only occur in a relational context where people feel safe." This type of yoga is an invitation to reclaim your body as your own. Emerson has more information on his website, traumasensitiveyoga.com.

Eye Movement Desensitization and Reprocessing (EMDR)

Although this method may seem a little odd—moving your eyes from side to side or hand-tapping as you recall images of a disturbing event—research shows EMDR really works for those struggling with trauma or difficult emotions. It's useful for those experiencing panic attacks or anxiety and those who have been sexually or physically abused.

Expressive Writing

Similar to journaling, expressive writing invites you to explore your thoughts and feelings that come up around a particularly traumatic or stressful event. Unlike journaling, however, the key is to write nonstop, without pausing to collect your thoughts, for ten to fifteen minutes. Think stream-of-consciousness journaling with a topic in mind.

Somatic Experiencing

Developed by trauma expert Peter Levine, Somatic Experiencing (SE) is a way of discharging stressful or traumatic emotions. Hala Khouri, a trauma-sensitive yoga teacher and practitioner of Somatic Experiencing, says that SE is about creating a space for people to tolerate the uncomfortable sensations and emotions associated with a traumatic event. "When we can tolerate the discomfort, we have the possibility of moving through it and releasing it, instead of going around it." SE is done with an SE-trained practitioner; to find one in your area, go to traumahealing.org.

Family Constellations

On the more esoteric side of things, we have Family Constellation work, developed by German psychotherapist Bert Hellinger in the mid-1990s, designed to help you understand, integrate, and heal your own trauma as well as your ancestral trauma. Done most often in group settings with a skilled facilitator, this work draws on a number of Western therapeutic models like Gestalt therapy, psychodrama, psychoanalysis, psychodynamic therapy, hypnotherapy, and family systems therapy, as well as traditional Zulu family beliefs. When done in a group, the participants act out the family issue of the person having the constellation, who is watching as family entanglements are revealed. For more information, see HealingTraumaCenter.com or hellingerpa.com.

HOW TO SHOW UP FOR YOUR PARTNER

The fertility journey is fraught with stress, which becomes much more acute when things feel like they're going terribly wrong. Miscarriages and failed IVFs are opportunities to bring couples closer instead of pulling them apart. Here are a few tips on how to be present with your partner through it all:

Don't take anything personally. If your partner has issues about her sexuality or her inability to get pregnant, it's not about you. Understanding this will help you be present without being defensive.

Communicate with your partner. Your job is to listen compassionately and patiently. No matter how many times she needs to process, no matter how many times he wants to talk about his fears or inadequacies. Through loving conversations, commit to discovering what each of you needs from the other to stay positive and to get through the hard times.

Reach out to others. What you both need is a good support system, beyond the two of you. Engage family and friends who love you, around whom you feel comfortable. People like that can have a positive effect on your mood and can, by their very presence, bring you closer together.

SEXUAL SECRET
Gently and lovingly transform trauma into empowerment using sexual healing with these Taoist techniques.

Acupressure points exist in many places in the body—the ears, feet, scalp, hands, and sexual organs being the most common ones. These microsystems correspond to the five elements of Chinese medicine and are used to treat the whole body. The basic idea is that we can create sexual healing by stimulating the different parts that correspond to the vagina and the penis. Taoists give sexual positions to heal different ailments because they believe that sexual energy can be used to heal our mind, body, and spirit and can thus connect us to the Divine. In heterosexual couples, penetration that brings the tip of the penis close to the cervix can create a heart-to-heart connection. You can also do sexual healing with or without a partner or with a partner of the same sex.

Try this: Touch an area that corresponds to one of the five elements that needs healing. For example, if you are frustrated, you might spend more time touching the part on the vagina or penis that corresponds to Liver energy. Experiencing pain in your genitals, maybe from trauma? Linger near the entrance to the vagina or the base of the penis, both of which are governed by Kidney energy. Or spend some time—either alone or with your partner—simply feeling your sexual energy and direct that energy into the parts of your body that need healing. Putting love into places that have experienced trauma can be a special part of a trusting relationship.

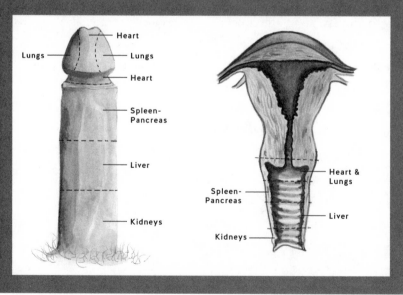

Establishing Sex-Positive Beliefs

Personal trauma, ancestral pain, and even cultural stigmas attached to sexual beliefs can result in shame and fear and an inability to enjoy sexual pleasure with the person you love. Case in point: A couple years ago I drove to a retreat with a woman from Ireland. Since I was writing a book on intimacy and fertility, she began to tell me about her relationship with her husband and their desire to have another child. They had been the best of friends—in fact, she said, they still were. But when bedtime rolled around, all she wanted to do was sleep. She felt terrible that she was rejecting her husband sexually, but she just didn't feel sexy and was too ashamed to talk about it. "You know," she confessed, "I grew up Protestant, and no one ever spoke about sex. There was a lot of shame around touching yourself or feeling any sexual feelings at all."

Other causes of shame and guilt can crop up during a couple's fertility journey, such as "I don't deserve to be a mom," "I can't get pregnant because I had an abortion when I was seventeen," or "I can't get my wife pregnant because I masturbated too often when I was a kid." When shame and guilt override desire, the inability to conceive can feel like a just punishment. It's easy to simply give up altogether.

It obviously doesn't have to be this way. As described above, there are many ways to heal from sexual trauma and to move beyond cultural opprobrium. But first it's important to understand what sex-positive beliefs are. According to the International Society for Sexual Medicine's (ISSM) website, the term *sex-positive* can be interpreted in different ways. "For most, it involves having positive attitudes about sex and feeling comfortable with one's own sexual identity and with the sexual behaviors of others."[5] You may have grown up in a culture whose beliefs about sexuality don't align with your own, or you may have beliefs that are diametrically opposed to your partner's.

Sometimes the hardest thing to do is to talk about your own sexual beliefs and learn about your partner's—without judgment. But true intimacy depends on it; being able to enjoy sex without shame or awkwardness, a healthy and normal part of life, depends on it. The key to all sexual activity is honest communication and consent without pressure.

Commit to supporting each other. Of course, past sexual trauma can and often does show up in current relationships, so it's imperative that each partner provide a safe container for the other and show up for the other with love.

Explore cultural and familial messages. Spend some time considering the messages you received growing up. If they were overwhelmingly negative or confusing, see how it would feel to flip them to positive. There's a method in the ancient yoga texts called "cultivating the opposite." If you've been told that feeling turned-on is wrong or dirty, see what it feels like to *affirm* those feelings. Make positive declarations, such as "I feel connected, loved, and beautiful" or "I love giving and receiving pleasure."

Write a history of your own sexual experiences and fertility challenges. This exercise doesn't dwell on or judge any of your experiences. It's simply to help you understand where you've been, where you are now, and where you want to go. Begin with the age you were when you first remembered having sexual feelings, your first wet dream, your first sexual attraction, your first menstrual cycle, first intercourse, first time you tried to conceive, first miscarriage or abortion. With each one, jot down any concerns you had or how you felt about yourself.

JADE EGG PRACTICE

For thousands of years, women in the East have used jade eggs for everything from strengthening and toning the vagina and having a better sex life to recovering from childbirth, healing from physical or emotional trauma, and increasing their chances of getting pregnant.

Why Jade?

Jade is thought to enhance the body's own energy, assist fertility, support the heart chakra, and increase yin essence (blood flow and bodily fluids). Emotionally, it helps release irritability, soothes the mind, and encourages us to share our hearts with others. Buy only jade that is GIA-certified, that is, from the Gemology Institute of America, the world's foremost authority on diamonds, colored stones, and pearls.

Whom Does It Help?

Women who feel physically cut off from their genitals and experience pain (because of physical or emotional trauma), those whose vagina feels closed up or excessively tight, those who want to awaken their connection to their sexuality. Inserting the jade egg, with love and tenderness, can help build up the tissues so that intercourse will be less painful.

When Shouldn't You Use It?

Do not wear this egg continuously, contrary to what some websites tell you. Do not use it if you are menstruating, are already pregnant, have a vaginal infection or a sexually transmitted infection, or have an IUD inserted. If you are trying to conceive, stop using the jade egg after ovulation.

How Should You Use It?

Step one: Place the jade egg in a pot, cover it with water, and boil it for ten minutes to sterilize.

Step two: Remove the egg and let it cool completely.

Step three: Take a piece of unflavored, unwaxed dental floss the length of your arm (about twelve inches) and thread it through the hole; tie a secure knot at the narrow end of the egg. This is so you can take it out easily.

Any Other Caveats?

Yes, the jade egg will strengthen a weak pelvic floor and can help decrease pain during intercourse, but be aware that pain doesn't always mean your pelvic floor muscles are too loose or that they're too tight. According to physical therapist Dustienne Miller, of Boston-based Flourish Physical Therapy, pain can be a remnant of an old bladder or yeast infection even after the infection has cleared up because of the holding mechanisms we have in our body. If you're experiencing vaginal pain, Dustienne recommends you consult your ob-gyn and a women's physical therapist who specializes in the pelvic floor.

Releasing Stress

....

Be content with what you have;
rejoice in the way things are.
When you realize there is nothing lacking,
the whole world belongs to you.

—LAO TZU

JIM AND STAR HAD BEEN STRUGGLING to make a baby for two years. By the time Star came to me, she was stressed, depressed, and, as she pointed out between sobs, already forty years old. As a busy executive she worked more than fifty hours a week in a job she hated; in addition, she volunteered for four charity groups, which she loved. Star told me that she had done *everything* to get pregnant and, I must admit, the list was impressive. She exercised, took herbs and vitamins, followed a very strict diet, recorded her temperature scrupulously every morning, and even did regular ovulation kits. She scheduled vitamin IV drips recommended by her naturopath; she tried to get at least six or seven hours of sleep (which she admitted wasn't enough); she read books, consulted experts, did hypnosis, wore special fertility-enhancing jewelry, and had sex perfectly on schedule three times a week before they turned to assisted reproductive medicine. She rattled all this off, punctuating it with frequent sighing.

When Star and Jim didn't get pregnant after all this, they went the IVF route, but she was a poor responder to the drugs, usually making only one follicle that housed a single egg. So they cancelled IVF and turned to intrauterine insemination (IUI), but that wasn't successful either. All the tests confirmed that her hormone levels were fine and her husband's sperm parameters were normal. The doctor said her infertility was unexplained, and concluded it was a result of her advanced maternal age—definitely not the conclusion she was willing to accept.

So there we were, in my office. As a practitioner of Chinese medicine, I knew her pulses could clue us in to what was going on. The Chinese diagnosis, based on her pattern, was clearly Liver qi stagnation and some Kidney deficiency. That meant all of the frustration, shame, and anger she felt because she could not control her fertility outcome was compromising her wood element energy. When that happens, the Liver qi becomes stuck and the body's qi is not able to flow freely throughout the body—most critically, into her reproductive organs. I see this often with type-A people who don't know how to slow down or take time out to relax. Their adrenal glands (Kidney energy) are working overtime, churning out cortisol (a stress hormone) to keep up with an overly stimulated sympathetic nervous system. In the meantime, no blood flow is getting to the reproductive system, which has effectively shut down.

Star was in fight-flight-freeze mode, a normal nervous system response to a stressful situation. Think saber-toothed tigers from days of old or almost getting hit by a bus along a busy thoroughfare. When we're stressed, whether that stress is caused by an emotional upset or a physical condition, such as high blood sugar or inflammation, our brain's amygdala registers danger and sends the body messages to activate the sympathetic response. In addition to the heightened adrenal activity, all systems of the body we need in order to fight or flee, or freeze, are ready—everything we need to see and think clearly, move quickly, and fight, if we have to. All other systems shut down, including our reproductive organ function. Elevated cortisol levels signal that it is not safe to make a baby.

As Star and so many of my patients will attest, there's enough stress in daily life under normal circumstances, so adding fertility challenges to all that can feel like too much to handle. Stress can show up during fertility challenges in many ways.

FOR MEN

~ Inability to get an erection

~ Inability to ejaculate

~ Lack of sex drive

~ Depression

~ Inability to make sperm (spermatogenesis)

~ Resentment of partner

~ Feelings of not being able to "fix" the situation

~ Feelings of inadequacy

~ Guilt because his partner has to go through fertility treatments when it's his sperm that is not adequate

FOR WOMEN

~ Lack of sex drive

~ Inability to orgasm

~ Decrease in vaginal lubrication

~ Menstrual cycle irregularities (cortisol affecting the hypothalamus-pituitary axis, or HPA)

~ Depression

~ Withdrawal from life

~ Anger and jealousy

~ Body-loathing as fertility treatments can increase weight

~ Feelings of not being understood by partner

A 2014 study published in *Human Reproduction* found that higher levels of stress were associated with "a longer time-to-pregnancy (TTP) and an increased risk of infertility."[1] A saliva test can measure your stress cortisol levels, which should be lowest in the morning and highest at night. Depending on what those levels are, an acupuncturist, naturopath, or functional medicine practitioner can suggest specific herbs and supplements to regulate them. For cortisol levels that are high in the evening, for example, supplements such as phosphatidylserine may help, as well as adaptogenic herbs such as ashwagandha, rhodiola, and Siberian ginseng.

If, on the other hand, you have completely burned out your adrenal glands from chronic stress, you may need an adrenal glandular to nourish and normalize adrenal function. I recommend that you talk to your health-care practitioner first, who will steer you in the right direction.

HOW DO WE MANAGE STRESS AND GET BACK TO LOVING AND PLEASURE?

It's hard. Regardless of gender, age, race, or religious beliefs, fertility struggles can turn anyone into a hot mess, no matter how "together" they were when they started out. Luckily, various tried-and-true mindful practices, along with a healthy lifestyle, can help. If you approach the exercises in this chapter with an open heart and the intention to stay present, they can also help you in the bedroom. When we have compassion for our own shadow self, we can be more vulnerable and authentic with our partner. Of course, it's risky telling the truth about our emotions. It's hard to admit to your partner that your feelings might not be logical, that you don't want to make love because if you don't have sex, then you won't feel like a failure if you don't get pregnant. Hopefully, the practices here can reduce the stress you're both under and lead to greater self-acceptance and greater connection. Choose the ones you feel most comfortable exploring.

Vipassana (Insight Meditation)

Vipassana, which in Sanskrit means "to see things as they really are," is the most ancient form of Buddhist meditation. Also known as Insight Meditation, this practice can help us become aware of what we're thinking and feeling as it is happening without judging, dissecting, or holding on to any of it. For couples dealing with fertility, the unknown is scary; it's hard not to jump into the future, which only increases fear and longing. Vipassana keeps us anchored in the present moment.

Jack Kornfield, a Buddhist teacher, author, and the founder of Spirit Rock Meditation Center, offers a helpful way of approaching this practice, which he calls "naming the demons." When we acknowledge our emotions and name them, we can work with them in our practice. We can dive a little deeper and see what lives underneath our anger (could it be fear?) or our longing (inadequacy maybe?). I don't know a single couple trying to have a child who doesn't have a collection of strong, often confusing and contradictory emotions to choose from: anger, jealousy, fear, doubt, blame, craving, hope, love, anticipation. What are yours? Sit with your feelings as they arise—name them and allow them to teach you. One of my Buddhist teachers suggests we then acknowledge these arisings by saying, "And this, too."

Jealousy is a particularly pernicious demon for many of my patients. They tell me how hard it is for them to see family members, friends, co-workers, or even women walking by who are pregnant. It's even more difficult when they have to talk to them. And, then, of course, they are ashamed of feeling jealous in the first place, which makes it almost impossible to stay present or connect with the people they normally love being with. Insight Meditation allows for all of these feelings to arise, be acknowledged, and named. And if we can separate our feelings from the story they're attached to (*I'll never get pregnant; I'm too old; I can't stand being around my friends*), we can perhaps see them in a different light and eventually release them.

Though it's not meditation-specific, I found a 2012 study to be a validation of the practice of Insight Meditation. Subjects of this study who were afraid of spiders were introduced to a live spider, and the researchers had them do one of four things: label their emotions, reappraise their thoughts about the spider, distract themselves completely from having thoughts about the spider, or just be in the room with the spider. Those who were able to name how they felt had a greater reduction in their fear response.[2]

INSTRUCTIONS FOR BEING PRESENT, OR INSIGHT MEDITATION

1. Sit in a comfortable position. Begin by simply breathing in and out of your nose and noticing the nature of your mind. Many of my patients say they can't possibly meditate because their mind is much too active. Meditation is not about emptying your mind or even trying to control it. In Insight Meditation, you watch your thoughts and feelings as if they are going by on a movie screen.

2. Greet all of the thoughts and feelings that arise as if you are lovingly parenting a child. In fact, in this way you are spiritually re-parenting yourself. If your child was fearful, you wouldn't tell her to stop feeling that way. Chances are you would gently comfort her, acknowledge her feelings, and give her a hug, reminding her, "I am here." Can you show up for yourself in the same way? Think of this as good practice for real parenting.

3. Take some deep diaphragmatic breaths and arrive at where you are now; gently put aside the twenty things you need to do.

4. Notice how your body feels. Notice when your mind wanders—and yes, it will wander. Name what you feel and gently come back to your breath.

5. Practice for as long as you'd like—ten to thirty minutes. But don't force it. Remember, it's all about self-inquiry with kind attention.

Here's an experience I had that might help you understand the types of things that come up in meditation. One morning when I was meditating I became aware of an old familiar feeling in my stomach. I recognized it right away—we've been together since I was a little girl—and immediately went down the poor-me rabbit hole. What was underneath those feelings? Then I saw it: fear—fear of failure, fear of rejection—and I named it. As I did, I could feel the fear welling up in my body and I started to cry. I didn't try to hold on to the sensation; I didn't try to explain it or attach it to anything.

I simply sat with it. And then . . . as I continued to breathe, the tightness in my stomach relaxed, the fear dissolved, and love took its place.

With practice, we come into contact with the tenderness that lives inside. Rather than push our feelings down with a big NO, we can meet them with compassion. It's not easy sometimes, that's for sure. But it does get better with practice. Have you ever gone on a strenuous hike and you thought you'd never get to your destination? And then you wondered why you agreed to do it in the first place? But you finally make it, and the next time you try the hike it's a little easier. By the time you've taken the same hike ten times, it's a piece of cake.

Something like this happened to me a few years ago. I was staying up in the mountains and wanted to take a hike. The innkeeper told me to stay on the road until I got to a park—should take about thirty minutes, he said. So, the next morning, with too many layers on and my water bottle in hand, I started out. The road wound around and around, and the walk seemed to take forever. I kept going until finally I made it to the park. The sun sparkled on a large granite wall; I stood in silence watching a hawk circling overhead. It was beautiful and totally worth the climb. The next morning, I decided to do it again. This time I reached the park in what felt like no time at all. The first time we try something it can be a struggle, but the second time it can feel more comfortable, and with practice it becomes second nature. It is the same way with Insight Meditation.

THE COUNTING MEDITATION

My patients often get so wound up they have a difficult time lying on my table, even with the acupuncture needles in them in a treatment that's designed to calm the nervous system. In such cases I give them a counting meditation to do while they lie there (or for any other time they feel stressed). Calm, steady breathing calms the nervous system.

continues

1. Find a comfortable seated position or lie down, whichever is most comfortable.
2. Take a moment or two to simply breathe in and out of your nose, focusing on a gentle, extended exhalation.
3. Begin to count your breaths at the end of each exhalation, until you reach ten; then begin again.
4. When you notice you've lost the count, simply start over again at one. No big deal.
5. Practice as long as you wish—could be five minutes or up to thirty minutes.

FORGIVENESS PRACTICE

Sometimes we hold on to hurt, anger, or resentment toward our partner—or toward our own self—which prevents us from feeling connected in a loving way. Or perhaps we need to ask for forgiveness for ourselves because our words or actions were unkind. How can we make love when there is a part of ourselves that is disconnected and not open.

There are many ways to encourage forgiveness. The simplest, yet quite profound method comes from an ancient Hawaiian practice called *ho'oponopono*, in which you say, "I'm sorry, please forgive me, thank you, I love you."

A traditional Buddhist forgiveness practice goes like this:

To those whom I may have caused harm, knowingly or unknowingly, through my thoughts, words, and actions, I ask your forgiveness.

To those who may have caused me harm, knowingly or unknowingly, through their thoughts, words, and actions, I offer my forgiveness as best I am able.

For any harm I may have caused myself, knowingly or unknowingly, through my thoughts, words, and actions, I offer my forgiveness as best I am able.

Acupuncture

Acupuncture is a powerful treatment to reduce or manage stress, and more studies have shown its positive effect on depression and anxiety. It can get stuck energy unstuck and correct imbalances in the organs, including the reproductive organs, as well as the autonomic nervous system and the central nervous system. Acupuncture releases endorphins, the body's own feel-good hormones, and can also reset your menstrual cycle and lessen menstrual pain.

Yoga

Coming into your body can help you explore the places where you hold tension so that you can learn how to release it. Kiki Lovelace is a Forrest Yoga senior teacher and the owner of Innerstellar, a pilates and yoga studio in Berkeley, California. She says that by bringing the breath and your "finest-quality attention" to the sensations in your body, you "learn how to use your yoga practice to ease the locked-up or shut-down places inside." She adds that learning "how to make connections between your body pains and tweaks and dead spots and your emotional world is deeply empowering. You discover deep wells of compassion inside, which you can pour over your wounds so they can better heal, and you can walk free of their power over you. We call this 'walking your freedom road.'" Pranayama (conscious breathing) techniques and deeply restorative practices are also extremely helpful to release tension and reset the nervous system.

SEXUAL SECRET

This simple yoga move is guaranteed to diffuse any stress or difficulties you are having with each other.

Kia Miller is a yoga teacher (Vinyasa, Ashtanga, and Kundalini styles) who offers classes in the United States, India, and Europe. She shared this yoga *kriya* (techniques that purify the body, mind, and spirit), which Yogi Bhajan gave to Guru Singh when he and his wife were having problems.

Stand, facing away from each other, spreading your legs wide. Bending from the hips, release forward so that you are both looking at each other upside-down. From this wide-legged forward bend, begin to sing your complaints to each other. It's truly impossible not to laugh!

PARTNER BREATHWORK

My partner tells me that one of the ways he feels connected is to start and end each day with closeness. What better way to do this than by breathing together? Pranayama quiets the sympathetic nervous system and engages the parasympathetic response. There are various techniques, here is one:

1. Sit back-to-back and breathe at same rhythm, inhaling and exhaling together. This is called *sama vritti* pranayama (even regulated breathing), in which you inhale gently to a count of, say, three, four, or five—whatever count feels good to you both—and then exhale same number of counts.
2. Sit facing each other and do individual breathwork, such as alternate-nostril breathing (*nadi shodhana*), described in chapter 8, or bee breath (*bhramari*), which is one of yoga teacher Linda Sparrowe's favorite pranayama techniques for raising the energy and lessening anxiety. It pretty much drowns out any mental chatter that keeps you on edge.

Here's how to practice bee breath:

1. Sit facing each other in a comfortable position.
2. Breathe gently and fully for a few breaths as you settle in, letting go of any tension you are holding on to, especially in your face.
3. Close your ears with your thumbs and, very lightly, touch the inner corners of your eyes with your index fingers.
4. Place your middle fingers on outside of your nose, your ring fingers above your lips (just under the nostrils), and your pinky fingers below the lips.
5. Inhale through the nose, and as you exhale, buzz like a bee until the exhale is complete. Make the buzz more like a bee (low-to-medium pitch) and less like a mosquito.
6. Do this pranayama for five or six rounds, stopping if you become light-headed.

YOGA NIDRA

Yoga nidra, or yoga sleep, is a deeply restorative practice in which your body is in a state between wakefulness and sleep. This practice is helpful for fertility, according to Uma Dinsmore-Tuli, a yoga therapist, founder of the Yoga Nidra Network, and the author of *Yoni Shakti: A Woman's Guide to Power and Freedom through Yoga and Tantra.* She told me that infertility with no known cause may not make sense at the physical level, but could maybe "be explained on an intuitive level, or as some kind of deeper emotional issue, or even as something energetic that needs to move in ways that are quite subtle." Uma loves yoga nidra. "It's amazing," she says, "because you lie down and you listen and you drop into a state that allows you to connect with these other dimensions of being that we often don't have time for because people are so busy. People haven't got time for love or anything else that gives them joy." By doing yoga nidra, "people can come into touch with the deep feminine. You can't do it wrong." She told me that yoga nidra is also a wonderful practice for couples. You do it together by cuddling up, with your partner's heart facing the back of yours. (For more information and free yoga nidra downloads, go to the resources section at the back of this book.)

Sound Meditation

In a 2011 pilot study using functional MRIs, researchers discovered that chanting the mantra *om* dampens down the fight-flight-freeze response of the sympathetic nervous system and activates the parasympathetic rest-and-digest response. The investigation proposed that this happens because deep sonorous sound is one way to tone the vagus nerve, a major part of the parasympathetic nervous system.[3] When you have high vagal tone, it means your vagus nerve is good at regulating your body and you enjoy lower stress levels, less anxiety, more resilience, lower blood pressure, and better moods. Low vagal tone, on the other hand, is often to blame for PTSD, chronic pain, inflammation, and poor digestion.

Other ways to tone the vagus nerve:

~ Slow, rhythmic, diaphragmatic breathing, especially ujjayi pranayama.

~ Humming or chanting anything with deep tones

~ Washing your face with cold water

~ Meditating

~ Balancing the gut microbiome

~ Ear acupressure. There's a point you can press called "Shen Men," which is in the triangular part of your ear closer to the top. Feel around for the tender point. I often needle this point in acupuncture, which brings instant calming. You can do it at home by pressing on this point yourself. (See the resource section at the back of this book for more information on how to locate this.)

Emotional Freedom Technique

Emotional Freedom Technique (EFT), or "tapping," as it is often called, is similar to acupuncture, but without the needles. In this technique you use your fingertips to tap specific acupuncture points on your body while repeating an affirmation to yourself and paying attention to how you're feeling. The affirmation can be anything, such as *Even though I feel completely discouraged, I accept myself exactly as I am.* Tapping was developed as a way to relieve stress and anxiety, to unstick places where energy is held, and to provide comfort. (For more information on the history and practice of EFT and additional resources, go to www.Goe.ac.)

Reframing Your Experience

When my patients panic because they've "failed" once again to become pregnant, I remind them about the mystery and beauty of life and encourage them to reframe their experience to include embracing the unknown. What if your child knows exactly when and how she wants to be born? What if she is waiting because she knows the friends and support you'll have when she does finally arrive, the worldly climate, the season? There's so much we don't know, so much we can't control, that perhaps there is wisdom in trusting the mysteries of life, even when it all feels so hopeless.

And sure enough, they tell me, that's often the case. Situations arise for them and reinforce the idea that everything happens in the right time, as it's supposed to. As Taoist teacher Solala Towler points out in *The Tao of Intimacy and Ecstasy*, "The seed of change is inherent in any situation, just as in the yin/yang symbol, the seed of one concept is inherent in the other."[4]

Compassion

I once took a class called "The Meaningful Life," where attachment theory met ancient Buddhist meditation. The instructor, George Haas, gave us each a rubber bracelet that read, "I love you, keep going." I like this phrase because it reminds me that life is forever moving and changing. How I feel can change from day to day, even moment to moment. If you are struggling with your relationship, with fertility, or with finding some inner peace, I invite you to have compassion for yourself and for others in this journey of life: "I love you, keep going—one moment, one breath at a time." It then becomes easier to tap into what is present right now—the beauty in a sunset, the smell of a rose, the laughter of your true love, the ability of your body to practice yoga, the constancy of your breath . . .

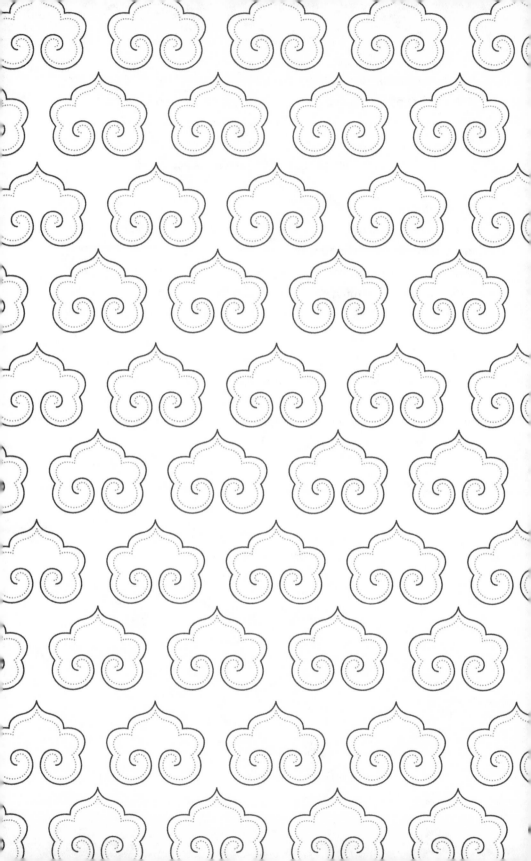

PART FOUR

Coming Together

Deepening Intimacy

....

I want soul sex, I need to taste your thought process,
together we can unravel riddles, the deeper the sweeter.

–UNKNOWN

BEING TRULY INTIMATE entails more than just jumping between the sheets. Couples must be open to listening intently and compassionately to the needs and desires of each other (the things said and the things left unsaid). But let's talk a bit about what that actually means.

Intimacy. *In-to-me-I-see.* Sounds like intimacy begins with yourself, doesn't it? It absolutely does. Think about it. It's pretty difficult to trust someone enough to share yourself fully if you don't feel worthy of that trust. Being intimate with someone means you allow them to see you for who you are at the deepest level of your being—not just the handpicked stories you prefer to share, but your authentic self. Of course, if you aren't comfortable with who you are, or if you're not even sure who you are or what you want or how to be happy, then intimacy will remain elusive.

When I was younger, I didn't have much self-confidence or even self-worth. I almost always chose men who I thought were more talented and accomplished than I was—one was a musician, another an artist, and a third a writer—and I lived vicariously through them. I felt inadequate around them until one day it dawned on me: *I could be a musician, an artist, or a writer, too, if I set my mind to it.* And so I did. I took up the guitar, expressed my art through dancing, and began to write. I have more to offer now because I feel fulfilled, which helps me show up to my partner feeling whole and worthy. I'm not saying that you have to take up the guitar, go to art school, or "do" anything else to feel good about yourself—that's an inside job. I am saying the art of self-love and the quest to discover your essential nature translate to freedom and a certain level of erotic energy. If you can love yourself unconditionally, including your perceived inadequacies, if you can embrace your whole body, flaws and all, you'll open yourself up to deeper intimacy.

I spoke to yoga teacher Kiki Lovelace about this very thing. She says, "To be truly intimate, you have to get this truth: your partner is not responsible for your health or happiness. Take responsibility for yourself, and make choices that help you step into your wiser self, choices that help you call your own spirit back to live fully in your body, so you don't have to feel so starving for nourishment or fulfillment from your partner all the time. Make healing and brightening choices for yourself, and you'll have so much more to offer your partner." Solid advice.

Intimacy isn't only about sex. It involves closeness, togetherness, affinity, attachment, affection, warmth, emotional and physical connection, openness, sensuous activity, and being comfortable sharing feelings. You can feel intimate with someone while wrapped up in a warm blanket, drinking hot chocolate, or belting out a song together during karaoke night and laughing uncontrollably. Being close can bring to light aspects of yourself you didn't even know were there and inspire you to discover aspects of your partner they weren't even aware of. Intimacy is all about getting to know yourself first and then committing to know your partner so well that you can tell when they are struggling and then listening and trying to help.

To fully open up sexually, you have remove the mask you're wearing and surrender to your partner. In other words, you must trust each other. Margo Anand, a tantra expert and the author of many books on the subject, says, "In an atmosphere of trust, you do not blame your partner for not fulfilling your desires. You accept the fact that in some ways you are different, yet recognize that you both bring precious gifts to the relationship that can make it nourishing and rewarding."[1]

Couples plagued with fertility issues either grow closer or fracture apart, and the key to the former is to find a way to make each other a priority, says Andrea Miller, founder of YourTango, a digital media platform dedicated to love and relationships. In her book *Radical Acceptance: The Secret to Happy, Lasting Love*, Miller says that to be successful in a relationship you have to accept and love your partner for who they are and not what you want them to be. When your partner does something that annoys you, you must "stop, reflect and introspect: get outside of [your] emotional reactions." She reminds us that "love is paramount no matter what form it takes."[2] Going one step further, I encourage my patients to focus on four intimacy essentials, or what I call the PECK model. Their homework is to look at each essential and see where they need to concentrate their attention, what might be missing in their relationship equation, and consider how they might reclaim it:

Passion: your desire and creativity; your ability to light the fire and awaken Eros

Exploration: your willingness to try different things, mix things up, and get to know yourself and each other

Communication: your ability to ask for what you want, talk to your partner about your feelings, and establish healthy agreements

Knowledge: your awareness of your body, what it needs to function well and to respond to your partner sexually; your ability to discern what to do and not do in your journey toward parenthood, what to ask doctors, what classes to take

INTIMACY AND BODY IMAGE

Sadly, but not surprisingly, one of the main reasons women avoid intimacy (especially sexual intimacy) is because they hate their bodies. I know my own story is not that different than that of millions of other women. I grew up in Los Angeles, where the media led us to believe that having the perfect body was everything. In high school I was always on a diet, determined to cram my muscular thighs into impossibly skinny jeans, forever comparing myself to girls skinnier than I would ever be.

As if the complicated relationship we have with the parts of our body others can see isn't enough, many men and women obsess over their private parts. Questions abound, like *Am I big enough to satisfy her? Am I wet enough? Are my vulva lips too long or too wide? How do I taste? How do I smell?* All of these questions can leave women and men too insecure to give and receive pleasure. Can we put those questions aside and instead ask: *How can I show my gratitude to my beloved? How can I love more deeply?*

Gratitude is a critical component in all relationships, and particularly important for women who are injecting themselves with fertility drugs that make them feel uncomfortable and sometimes even repulsed by their bodies. I attended an IVF transfer of supermodel Chrissy Teigen, whose husband, the Grammy Award–winning singer John Legend, was on tour at the time. Right after the transfer, they FaceTimed. I was moved to tears when I heard him say to Chrissy, "Thank you so much for doing all this. I really appreciate you and I love you." I must say, I have attended many, many IVF transfers and I have rarely witnessed a husband express gratitude for all his wife has to go through with medical intervention. The lyrics in his song "All of Me" convey it best: "All of me loves all of you."

GRATITUDE PRACTICE

1. Choose a physical aspect of your partner that you appreciate and lovingly comment on it. It could be anything, such as "I love the shape and feel of your belly. It's so soft and sensual." Or perhaps, "I love your chest and I can't stop running my fingers through your chest hairs."
2. Choose actions you appreciate from your partner and express your gratitude: "I love that you're so patient with me." "I really appreciate it when you make me dinner." "Thank you for taking such good care of me when I feel so awful."

3. Now, take that appreciation to another level and compliment each other on your sexual parts. You might say something like: "I love the way you taste." "We are such a perfect fit." "The inside of your lips are a beautiful color." "Your penis is the perfect shape and size for me and gives me a lot of pleasure."

I know, I know, it'll seem a bit awkward at first, but it gets easier with practice. I promise.

Gratitude softens us to receive love and feel a sense of belonging, which is our biological imperative. When we feel appreciated, we feel seen. But there is nothing quite like the internal flame that lights up when we look into the eyes of another, see their soul, and fall in love. I attended a workshop called "Healing the Healer," which began with my friend sharing a four-minute Amnesty International video, *Look Beyond Borders*. The video showed refugees from all over the world who were asked to pair off and look into each other's eyes for four minutes. This exercise was based on the work of psychologist Arthur Aron, best known for his work on intimacy, who discovered that four minutes of gazing into each other's eyes can bring two people closer. The short film reaffirmed that when we come to a situation with our hearts open, love spills out, and we connect soul-to-soul—there is no separation.

Of course, that discovery would hardly surprise many spiritual practitioners who are used to exercises that invite them to gaze into each other's eyes. After all, the eyes aren't called "the windows of the soul" for nothing. I once went to a White Tantric Yoga workshop in New Mexico, where more than two thousand people gathered to practice yoga, chant, and connect to their higher power. We did a lot of eye-gazing—sometimes for more than thirty minutes at a stretch. While we were looking into a partner's eyes, the teacher gave us powerful kriyas to purify the body, mind, and spirit; showed us specific mudras (hand positions) to hold; led us in chants; and instructed us not to break eye contact—all for anywhere from thirty-one to sixty-two minutes. Even though my arms felt like they were falling off and I really wanted to stop, I persevered because I didn't want to let my partner down. We changed partners several times and repeated the exercise, and every time I looked into the eyes of the person across from me, no matter who it was, I fell in love—every time! Afterward I understood why the teacher cautioned us not to make any radical decisions based on these exercises—the intimacy factor of gazing into a person's eyes for that long was incredibly high.

When was the last time you sat quietly and gazed into the eyes of your beloved? If it's been awhile, try this experiment for four minutes.

EYE-GAZING PRACTICE

1. Pick a space that resonates with both of you. You may wish to light a candle or turn the lights on; it's best without fluorescent lights.
2. Sit across from each other in a comfortable position. Prop yourself up on pillows, if this feels more comfortable. Holding hands is fine.
3. Take a moment to close your eyes and simply breathe, feeling grounded and calm. When you're ready, you can squeeze each other's hands and open your eyes.
4. Softly gaze into each other's eyes. Some people say it's easier to stare into the left eye—that's our receptive side—but it's also okay if you toggle between the left and the right.
5. Maintain this contact for four minutes, if possible. Notice what feelings come up. Notice the urge to look away. Be aware of all the sensations that arise.
6. Close by giving each other a deep, connected embrace.

EYE-GAZING DURING LOVEMAKING

Once you're comfortable gazing into each other's eyes for at least four minutes, you can try it when you make love. Keep the lights on soft and low, but enough so that you can see each other. Psychologist David Schnarch, a sex and marital therapist and the author of *Passionate Marriage: Keeping Love and Intimacy Alive in Committed Relationships*, advocates looking at your partner during foreplay, kissing, and orgasm. You may find it awkward at first, but it really can be powerful to notice—really notice—the person you are making love to. You certainly don't have to look at each other the whole time; maybe you will both decide to open your eyes during foreplay—or only during orgasm. I know when I first tried it during an orgasm I found it difficult to be seen like that. But then I simply let go. Once I did, I connected so deeply with my partner I wasn't even conscious of having my eyes open. Of course, there's also something quite wonderful about closing your eyes and receiving. Try them both—or alternate between the two as you make love.

THE POWER OF TOUCH

After gazing into each other's eyes for as long as you wish, it might be time to explore each other with loving touch. The dance of intimacy is knowing at each moment what your partner needs by reading the signs they offer you or by listening to what they like. Become an explorer of your partner's intimate landscape. It doesn't matter how long you've been together, greeting your beloved as though you were touching for the very first time is quite exquisite. Approach each other with the express desire of giving pleasure. This helps you break out of predictable patterns, where you're doing the same thing sexually over and over again. See what happens when you bring a new awareness to your lovemaking.

Some say that women are like rose petals, slowly opening their love palace to those who are patient. Others describe men as more like a furnace—their fire burns strongly, but they need a woman, who is the kindling that ignites that fire.

INTIMATE TOUCH EXERCISE

Before you get started, here are a few suggestions. Feel free to come up with your own:

1. Ask your partner if there are any places they would not like to be touched.
2. Always ask for feedback to make sure you're not doing anything that doesn't feel good.
3. Begin by exploring their body with your hands, which can be very powerful.
4. Your partner might like to be blindfolded when receiving your touch. Ask first.
5. Have your partner lie down on their back.

Light Touch

1. Start caressing your partner's face with a light touch, like the feel of a rose petal on the face. You can even incorporate actual rose petals if you like. As tantra teacher Dawn Cartwright says, "Put love in your fingertips."
2. Caress each area for about five strokes: forehead, eyebrows, eyes, cheeks, lips, and the ears—all the way to the neck.

Squeezing Touch

1. Gently guide your fingers from your partner's head down to the left side of their body. Begin by squeezing the top of the shoulders—the trapezius muscle between the shoulders and the neck—and then move down the arm and to the hand, using the same squeezing motion. This should wring out any tension in the muscles. Repeat on the right side of body.
2. Continue with this squeezing technique on the hips, all the way down the leg, and on to the left foot.
3. Repeat on the right side of body.

Finger Pad Touch

1. Using the pads of your fingers like raindrops, start at top of the left shoulder and move down the left arm into the hand. Repeat on right side of body.
2. With that same raindrop motion and pressure, return to the left side and start at the hips and move down the leg and into the left foot.
3. Repeat on the right side.

Feather Touch

1. Next, using a gentle touch, as soft as a feather, begin to softly brush the chest, moving down the torso all the way to the genitals.
2. Make sure to circle the nipples and the genitals and maybe gently brush them. Linger in areas when you notice your partner's breathing changes.

COMMUNICATE, COMMUNICATE, COMMUNICATE

It's lovely to have nonverbal means of communication, like eye-gazing and sensual touch, but what if you need more time to talk with your partner to feel connected, or what if your beloved feels especially cared for when you send him or her "just because" presents? That's okay, too. You may have different ways of receiving and responding to love, says Gary Chapman, author of The Five Love Languages. Chapman says, "How do we meet each other's deep emotional need to feel loved? If we can learn that and choose to do it, the love we share will be exciting beyond anything we've ever felt."[3] It's good to remember that we are not all wired the same. Taking time to understand your partner's needs—and communicating your own—is one way to light the fire of the mind and invite passion in.

HONESTY IS THE BEST POLICY

For more than ten years I have been attending a family camp where I've noticed one couple who seem to be totally into each other. I knew they had two daughters in their twenties who also attend the camp. How could they still be so much in love? I just had to ask "What's your secret?"

"We are brutally honest with each other," was the answer. They don't harbor resentments that can siphon off sexual energy and connection. When we are honest with each other we can share our fears around intimacy without being rejected. I knew a guy who liked to keep his button-down shirt on whenever he made love. His partner thought that was a little strange, but when he admitted that he didn't like to be naked on the top because he was ashamed of his chest, which he thought was too big, she completely understood. With her understanding he was able to shed his shirt and feel better about how he looked.

HONESTY

Even if you become fluent in each other's love language, when it comes to the bedroom you may still have a difficult time asking for what you want sexually. Emily Morse, a sex and relationship expert and the host of the podcast *Sex with Emily*, agrees. "We are so afraid of asking for what we want or even talking about sex," she told me. "It all goes back to shame, vulnerability, and sexual trauma—and all these things can block us. Ultimately we are afraid we won't be loved." For many couples, when they add baby-making sex to the mix, exploring the intimate connection of communicating what they want and need gets shoved aside in favor of expediency.

Here are a few techniques that may help you get the conversation started; see what works for you and your partner.

Take the conversation out of the bedroom. Sex can be a difficult subject to navigate in the best of circumstances. So do yourself a favor and save the awkward conversation about what you like and what you don't for outside the bedroom—over coffee, over dinner, in the living room, in the kitchen . . . any neutral territory where you feel comfortable having a meaningful conversation is best. Keep it light, nonjudgmental, and loving.

Always start with something positive and use "I" statements.
No one likes to be told that the way they make love needs
improvement. So appreciate first. Things such as "I love the way
your hands caress my body; it feels so sensual and relaxing." And
then instruct. "Lately, though, I've been having a bit of a problem
climaxing and I'm not sure why. I started playing around with a little
self-pleasuring and discovered a new way to touch my clitoris that
really works. May I show you?"

Bring in new techniques you've read about. Tell your partner
you've read about a new technique you're dying to try and then
show your partner what it involves. Let him or her know you'd
like to explore different ways of touching each other's genitals to
discover what you both really like—light, hard, flicking, on the
G-spot, more time on the clitoris but only rub the hood—things
like that. A man might like you to try a twisting motion on his
penis using both hands.

Use specific wording to direct them. Higher, lower, faster, slower,
more pressure, less pressure, just right. If your partner is changing
it up when you want it to stay the same, you can say, "That feels
great, can you do that a little longer?" Too fast? Then try "Slow
down, I want to savor every moment of this." Too gentle? "Harder,
please." And when you are wanting a tender, softer touch? "I would
love it gentle today."

Show instead of tell. If talking about what you like and don't like
doesn't work for you, guide your partner's hand to where you
want to be touched. When they get it right, be sure to let them
know how good it feels. Positive reinforcement, like groans of
ecstasy, works miracles.

Learn together. Another way to take ego out of the conversation is
to encourage your partner to read books or watch educational sex
videos with you. It's fun to discuss what you've seen or read—and
maybe even practice a few of the suggestions. (See chapter 14 for
some things to try.)

Keep trying. Yes, these conversations and bedroom change-ups can sometimes be awkward and anxiety-producing. But if you both commit to opening up without assigning blame or shame, they can have a positive impact on your intimate connection.

PLAY THE THREE-MINUTE GAME

When two people with different sexual needs, wants, and desires try to communicate, everything can get botched up. One partner can be doing what they think the other person wants and the other person may or may not want it. For example, Don often squeezes Emily's breast rather hard because he thinks Emily likes it that way. Emily doesn't like it at all, but she doesn't say anything because she thinks Don gets turned-on squeezing her breasts that way. Chiropractor and certified sexological bodyworker Betty Martin offers the 3-Minute Game, created by life coach Harry Faddis, to help couples clarify what truly works for them. She gives them two questions they can take turns asking each other:

How do you want me to touch you for three minutes?

When your partner asks this question, you can respond by saying things like you'd like your face caressed or your back massaged or your nipples kissed. And you can even change the ask midway through.

How do you want to touch me for three minutes?

When your partner asks this question, always respond by asking permission before you touch. "May I play with your hair?" or "lick your ear" or "nibble your toes?" Your partner has the right to say no, of course.

Besides having fun, which Dr. Martin says is the main reason for this game, couples can use it as a way to learn to negotiate touch and levels of intimacy based on giving and receiving and doing and being done to. The 3-Minute Game, which you can download at BettyMartin.org, works nicely for couples trying to conceive because it helps them base their time together on pleasure instead of necessity. Touching becomes fun again.

INTIMACY DURING ASSISTED REPRODUCTION

Just because you're going through IVF or IUI, and intercourse is off the table, doesn't mean intimacy has to be. Spend time together—watching movies, playing board games, taking bike rides or walks, cuddling, massaging each other. Give yourselves a break from your fertility discussions. Janet, a patient of mine, told me that she and her husband always hang out on Saturdays. During their IVF they make it a point to do fun things together—visiting museums, walking on the beach, exploring a new neighborhood or town nearby. What they don't do is mention their fertility journey at all.

Share Your Sexual Fantasies with Each Other

How do you tell your partner your sexual fantasies without feeling judged or without making her or him feel inadequate? Because our culture or religious upbringing can create taboos around sexual fantasies, it can be tricky to confess that we have them and even harder to admit we'd like to explore them. Of course, not all fantasies are things we want to play out. Watching porn with crazy, way-out sex scenes may excite us, but that doesn't mean we're eager to have those very same experiences ourselves.

According to Celina Criss, PhD, a certified sex coach and self-described "pleasure advocate and kink specialist" based in Munich, Germany, "We first have to know it's okay to fantasize and then we have to figure out what our fantasies are, so we can put them into words," she says. "They don't have to sound coherent. Some people fantasize in colors and there is no specific script. Some blurt it out all at once, others feel safer over text messages, and some let the fantasy out drip by drip." For example, Dr. Criss told me there can be role-playing like, "I would like you to be the chef, and I will be the lobster, meet me in the bathtub in ten minutes and bring a wooden spoon."[4] My friend Marc told me that sex, for him, is sometimes about "elevating spiritually," but other times he likes the pure animal nature aspect of it. Obviously, communication is important, especially if you are going to be parents. There doesn't have to be a *right* fantasy. You want to be completely yourself wherever you are. In fact, if you are trying to conceive, the biggest fantasy you might have is becoming parents!

Acts of Devotion

So you have taken care of yourself, appreciated your partner, done some eye-gazing, touched your partner's body, figured out your love language, and asked for what you want. All of this is a way of devoting yourselves to each other, finding ways to love fully and deeply, even when you're faced with challenges like infertility, which threaten to break your hearts and drive a wedge between you. Jai Uttal, a Grammy-nominated musician and singer, is a Bhakti yogi, someone who sings kirtan (devotional chants), meditates, pays homage to the deities, and is devoted to the Divine and to his guru, Neem Karoli Baba. Jai also has the most beautiful relationship with his love, Nubia Teixeira, a yoga teacher and the founder of Bhakti Nova Dance. I asked him what his secret to a lasting relationship and intimacy was.

"I don't have any secrets. I've been in several really destructive relationships, but when I met Nubia, everything changed. Well, for one thing, I got sober. But more than that I felt, for the first time, that it was safe to be afraid. I could be needy and dependent and attached. I am—all the things that our modern-day philosophers say are detriments to 'real' love. But I hear and read and remember the stories of [the Hindu god and goddess] Krishna and Radha—their ecstatic bliss, their jealousy, their complete attachment to each other, their anger when the love isn't reciprocated— all of that. And then I read and hear and remember the love of Sita and Rama, who gave up *everything* to be together, and in the end chose separation to increase their longing for each other. Anyway, they are my models. The rest is grace. I'm afraid of intimacy and not very good at it, but I refuse to stop trying."

Relationships give us many blessings, and a baby is just one of them. Many people work so hard at making a baby that they forget that the loving connection they once shared with their partner is often what created the desire for a child in the first place. The invitation now is to remember to care for yourself and to care for each other, which can help you renew the bonds of love between you. To quote Charlie Chaplin, "Your naked body should only belong to those who fall in love with your naked soul."

SEXUAL SECRET

The Inner Smile is a Taoist practice guaranteed to bring a smile to your heart.

This Taoist meditation invites us to smile to our body. I've extended it to include the person you love as well.

1. With your eyes closed, visualize your own body; see your smiling face, and then take that energy in through your third eye and direct it to all of your body parts, including your reproductive and sexual organs. Notice how you feel.

2. Now, visualize an image of someone who loves you. See their smiling face. And just like you did for yourself, bring in that energy through your third eye and move it through your whole body. With your eyes still closed, feel what you feel. Can you smile, too?

3. I also love doing this meditation with my beloved. Stand or sit facing each other and with your eyes closed, feel their smiling energy and allow it to penetrate your entire being, moving through all parts of your body and lingering in your heart and down into your pelvis.

When I hear my inner critic judging my body, I switch to the image of my partner smiling in front of me—a reminder to put my critical voice aside and focus on gratitude and kindness for my body and all that it does. This can be very effective at letting go of the shame that lives within—particularly in our sexual parts—which can prevent us from not only being intimate, but letting go to orgasm.

14

Foreplay: The Sweet Seduction

....

CONTRARY TO WHAT MANY OF MY MALE PATIENTS BELIEVE, foreplay isn't something that happens in the first thirty seconds of lovemaking. It really is an enticement to sacred sex that begins with morning kisses, silly or meaningful ways of interacting, sweet acts of kindness, and brief erotic connections throughout the day. Lack of sensual foreplay is one of the most common complaints I get from my female patients, especially those trying to get pregnant.

My patient Rachel and her husband Phil are perfect examples of what I mean. When they came to see me, Rachel did the talking while Phil sat a safe distance away, fumbling with the zipper on his sweatshirt and barely making eye contact with either of us. "We are in the midst of fertility hell," Rachel said. "We've had no success doing Western treatments for the last two years." She was hoping for a second opinion from me about their treatment options. She was approaching forty and had never been pregnant. He was in his late thirties. Their official diagnosis: unexplained infertility.

We talked about energy, digestion, sleep, emotional well-being, hormones. According to both of them—and their doctor's report—everything was normal. It all looked good to me, too, until we got to the sex part. "Do you know how to time intercourse to maximize conception?" I asked. She gave him a quick look, which I interpreted as, "Is it okay for me to tell her about our sex life?" He didn't respond. Rachel continued. "We do. We have sex once a month during the fertile time, but not much more than that. I mean we're really busy—we work a lot—and this whole fertility thing has really stressed us both out." We talked a bit more, but her husband wasn't so keen on contributing. After a bit, Rachel said she'd get an acupuncture treatment and suggested to Phil that they could meet up afterward.

When I got Rachel alone in the treatment room, I asked her frankly about their sex life. She told me that sometimes intercourse is painful upon entry. She was worried that her estrogen was too low, but I had seen her blood tests and reassured her that her estrogen was in the normal range. Does it stay painful as intercourse goes on? "No," she said, "that part's good." Maybe dryness is causing the pain? No problem there, either. "Okay, I just have to ask," I said, "do you think there's enough foreplay?" "Foreplay? Hardly. These days we just do it to get it done. What he thinks of as foreplay is a little rub on each breast, a few kisses, and off we go. Or should I say off *he* goes!"

Rachel is pretty typical of the women I treat—high-powered executives who take on a largely masculine or yang role in their day-to-day lives. They're in charge, managing others, making decisions, moving at a fast pace from the time they leave the house until the moment they get home. And, then, of course, they jump into home life, which has its own challenges and chores. By the time evening rolls around, many of these women say they're too exhausted to even think about sex, unless it's during their fertile window—and then they need to make things happen right away.

My male patients admit that the sense of urgency is confusing to them. And frankly, they like foreplay, too, and contrary to what some women think, "it's not only about grabbing onto a guy's cock and balls," says psychologist Adam Sheck. "Men want to be touched, they want to feel appreciated. And—this is important—men are aroused by the process of arousing their partner."

Sheri Winston is a sexuality teacher, nurse-midwife, gynecological nurse practitioner, and the author of *Women's Anatomy of Arousal: Secret Maps to a Buried Pleasure*. She admitted to me that she has a problem with the word *foreplay* because "it gives you the idea that [what's happening] is not important, it's a prelude, an appetizer, and the real deal is intercourse." The whole act of making love should be an erotic encounter from beginning to end. Winston teaches a workshop called "Pussies and Puppies at Play." In the workshop she reminds men that if they want to pet a pussycat, they can't just go up to and grab it. "You have to attune to the pussy's signals and go as fast as it tells you to go," she says. "If you jump ahead and try to pet her tummy when she's not ready, it'll take twice as long to get her to relax. It's an animal thing." Puppies, on the other hand, she says, are generally simpler. "If you scratch a dog on its ear for ten seconds and then spend twenty seconds rubbing its back, it will roll over right away—eager and enthusiastic—and want you to rub its tummy." What Winston is driving at is that a man's sex center resides in his sex organs and his brain; for women, sexual energy depends first on connection, environment, story, context—and then begins to flow through thinking, communicating, feeling, and then finally moves into the genitals. Love takes time. Of course, these are generalizations, but certainly with my patients I find quite a bit of truth to them.

In fact, Masters and Johnson as well as Alfred Kinsey, pioneers in sexual research, reported years ago that it takes about twenty-one minutes of foreplay (or longer) for a woman to become aroused and have an orgasm. Winston says that in her experience it takes women even longer—thirty to forty-five minutes to get the mind and body in a deep state of arousal and activate all parts of the erectile network.

While becoming proficient at different ways of pleasuring is important, technique means nothing unless you put your whole heart into it. Sure, you can technically learn how to stimulate your partner with just your fingers, but if you're distracted and only going through the motions, your partner will feel it and it won't be a turn-on. Put some soul into your loving.

Think of foreplay as romance, seduction, gentle exploration, a way of creating trust and intimacy. Of course, myriad ways exist to instigate and enhance sexual excitement. Here are a few to investigate; obviously, when you commit to practicing, you'll find the ones that resonate with you and your love.

ALL-DAY FOREPLAY

There are all kinds of books to read, films to watch, and workshops to take to help you get you and your lover excited. But the most important lesson for all couples to learn is this: seduction begins in the morning. It truly is the little things that create connection and make a difference. One woman I know brings her girlfriend coffee every morning in bed; they get their morning started by lounging together, talking about nothing particularly consequential. Another woman told me she wakes her boyfriend up with a kiss, announcing that he's the sexiest person she knows. My partner often sends me special quotes he knows I'll appreciate—even if some are a bit corny. One morning I woke up to see "I love you" written in lipstick across my mirror. I thought of that all day. These days you can send a short audio or video that will make your partner smile. But remember, cybersex won't get you pregnant.

Make a Meal Together

There's something so wonderful about working together as a team to create a nourishing meal, even if you can't cook. It's a bonding moment that heightens the senses of smell, touch, and taste. Make a platter of fertile-friendly foods—a joyful way of eating to conceive (see "Sexy Foods" in chapter 7). Of course, if you need inspiration, there's always *Iron Chef*.

GET YOUR GROOVE ON—TOGETHER

Biodanza, a series of movements put to music, is designed to keep you fully present with each other. I had an opportunity to experience the power of it on a retreat in Prague. The teacher, Niraj, led us in a series of movements that involved intimate contact. As the music flowed, I got swept up in the rhythms, drumbeats, ebbs and flows, ups and downs, and fast and slows of the dance. Even in a class setting it all felt so intimate. I asked Niraj later what intimacy meant to him, and he said, "It's the simple act of looking into someone's eyes and remaining there, accessing emotions through their eyes and not getting thrown off by whatever is going on with them but instead being moved by it. For me, intimacy has a physical component, of course."

Niraj shared with me the following three exercises and music selections, which may facilitate a greater connection with your partner. Fortunately, you don't have to be a dancer to do them. Each exercise takes about three minutes or so. First, choose an appropriate piece of music. Choose something melodic and romantic, rather than percussive or rhythmic; with or without words. And then, begin.

Accompaniment of the head (music suggestion: "Because," by the Beatles): One person stands behind the other and places their hands lightly on either side of their partner's head—not too strongly as to inhibit movement, but not too lightly as to be an ephemeral presence. The front person rotates the head gently in one direction, giving a gentle stretch that should stay within the boundaries of a pleasant or, better yet, a pleasurable experience. The second person simply accompanies the movement, giving containment and safety/security for the other person to let go and surrender. At the close of the music, the back person rests their hands on the shoulders of the front person and they take a deep breath together. Repeat, switching places.

Accompaniment of arms (music suggestions: "Moments of Pleasure," by Barbra Streisand, or "Common Threads," by Bobby McFerrin): Same as before, one person stands behind the other. This time the front person places their hands on their heart first and then does an expressive dance using just the hands and arms (i.e., body, trunk, and legs stay still). Person in back follows the movement of this "dance" by lightly resting their arms on the front person's, accompanying their movement, wherever and however it's expressed. Both parties rest their hands on their heart at the conclusion of the music and breathe deeply together before switching places.

Accompaniment of the pelvis (music suggestion: "Muito," by Caetano Veloso): One behind the other, as above, this time the one in front circles the hips, making a figure eight, and rocks back and forth in a sensual "this gives me pleasure" movement. Explore all the ways you can feel good while being accompanied from behind by a witnessing presence. The dancer may place the hands of the accompanier on their hips. Then switch places.

Shower or Take a Bath Together

I love those special scrubbing mitts that make me feel like I'm having a spa treatment. Hot and steamy! Add some yummy-smelling natural scrubs or soaps, but remember to not soap your vagina.

Send a Video of Yourself

Make a short video of your sexy self and send it to your partner during the day with loving or naughty words.

Make Sweet Music Together

Is it true that musicians swoon their lovers with song? Then why not sing together or accompany each other on guitar, piano, harmonium, or any other instrument you love. Not musically inclined? Not to worry. A friend of mine and her partner played DJ for each other: she chose a song from her iTunes list that reminded her of something they'd done together; her partner reciprocated by choosing one of her own. Or there's always the advice given by the Kama Sutra: produce music by striking glasses of water.

Put It on the Calendar

I know, I know. Scheduling sex doesn't sound very . . . well, sexy. But you can make it fun by sending him or her a text with a red heart and instructions: "Be home at 7." I even read where one woman left a trail of chocolate kisses on the floor leading to the bedroom, where a heart shape in rose petals was decorating the bed.

Role-Play

Play like it's a first date, where you don't know each other. Meet at a bar, museum, farmer's market, and flirt like you're picking each other up. Or dress up in a costume of your choice and act out a scene as a doctor/nurse, police/victim—anything goes that you mutually decide on.

Bring a Little Play into the Bedroom

If a woman requires at least twenty minutes to get aroused, then her partner needs to get creative. The Kama Sutra details sixty-four acts that stimulate erotic desire prior to intercourse. They include embraces, caresses, kisses, stretching out against each other, sighs, bites, scratches, and light blows (not suggesting that you literally strike a blow to your partner). Some couples get really turned on by the more explicit practices of BDSM (bondage/discipline, sadism/masochism). If you do decide to play with whips, floggers, paddles, or any other BDSM tools, go slow and make sure you get some advice either from a professional or a website. If you are planning on role-playing with dominance and submission, negotiate the parameters first, and always have a safe word in case you want to stop.

Picnic

Pack a picnic and head to a secluded spot, perhaps one that holds special meaning for the two of you. Read poetry aloud to each other—love poems preferred!

Body Painting

Use nontoxic paints or maybe foods like berries or chocolate syrup (dark, of course), and decorate your partner's naked body (sorry, whipped cream is not on the fertility diet). Use a variety of brushes, sponges, and other painting tools to create a human art project. Paint whiskers and spots on your partner to make them into a jaguar. Use rub-on tattoos or make your own. Have fun and be creative.

Play Games

Play a good old-fashioned card game like poker (the strip variety, of course). Or check out couples games to order online. Be forewarned, however: I made the mistake of Googling adult games and got a whole list of porn games instead, which wasn't what I had in mind. But you never know what will work to get things going.

Leave Sexy Notes

Leave a sexy note in his pocket or affixed to the bathroom mirror, describing an exciting surprise that awaits when he returns home.

Watch a Sex Video or Read Erotica Together

If you don't know what your fantasies are, Celina Criss, the German pleasure advocate and "kink specialist" mentioned earlier, suggests going to Goodvibes.com, an online sex shop that has a selection of books on erotica, or check out the Center for Sex and Culture (sexandculture.org) for judgment-free education, a media archive, and other cool resources for those across the sexual gender spectrum.

Whispers in the Dark

Just the act of whispering in your lover's ear can be a great turn-on. My patient Terri loves to whisper in her partner Linda's ear, offering up her favorite fantasy or giving her little hints of what she'd like to do next.

Create a Bag Full of Sex Toys

Explore new ways to enhance pleasure by putting together a bag of sex toys and asking your partner to close their eyes and pick one to use. I once attended a fortieth birthday party where we got to break open a piñata. What came out of that papier-mâché donkey? A bunch of sex toys, of course! Read further for some more ideas about what to put in your piñata.

THE ART OF SENSUAL STIMULATION

Sensuality is the doorway to sexuality. It's important to remember that erogenous zones aren't limited to the genitals. Explore the whole body before you move down to the main attraction.

Touch for Women

There are endless possibilities to explore in a sexual relationship with a woman. The clitoris isn't all she wrote. Remember the vestibular bulbs of erectile tissue we talked about in chapter 1? Sometimes touching all around this area can arouse a woman. Some women like a light touch around their anal opening, a technique called "rimming." (Caution: fingers that play in this area are not to be inserted into the vagina.) Explore all the areas of the body with the fingers and tongue to find what gives your partner pleasure. By taking the time to do this, you open the possibility for more pleasure and greater connection.

RHYTHM AND PRESSURE: Have you thought much about how you like your clitoris stimulated? Tapping on the hood of the clitoris, do you prefer a slow, fast, or variable speed? Play your clitoris and vagina like a musical instrument, varying the tempo and the intensity. Perhaps you like a pattern like 1 and 2 and 3, with a pause and repeat? Or a longer pause to build up excitement. Or even a rhythm so fast that your body begins to vibrate. If you already have a rhythm and tempo that sends you into orgasm, don't change it; instead, alert your partner—by moaning or possibly through words like "Yes, yes, don't stop now!" Advice to partners: stay consistent when a woman is climaxing.

Besides paying attention to the rhythm of touch—and sharing the results of your "research" with your partner—experiment with pressure and pulsation. You may decide that you like gentle pressure that gradually builds up, teasing the clitoris. Most women don't like the head of the clitoris touched in the beginning because it is very sensitive. They prefer touching around the clitoris in more of a pulsing, vibrating, stroking pattern.

ORAL SEX: Of course, all the explorations of touch you've done on yourself with your fingers can also work extraordinarily well by using your partner's tongue. Many couples, especially lesbian couples, love going down on each other. But others, especially hetero couples, may experience some awkwardness at first or have body-image issues to work through. The fact is, many of us were raised in families or cultures where we learned that our bodies—and their fluids, sounds, and smells—are disgusting and should never be shared with anyone else. If that was your experience, and all this talk about oral sex makes you feel slightly queasy, be patient. You may want to explore your own pleasuring to help you get more comfortable with your body and its desires. (Review chapter 5.)

And partners, don't forget to let your beloved know how lovely her whole body is, including her vagina and vulva. I can pretty much guarantee she'll appreciate the compliment and open up more to you. And seriously, slow down. It takes patience and persistence to arrive at pleasure, so don't be in a hurry to get to the finish line. One more piece of advice, this one from Rachel Venning, a self-described "sexpert" and the author of *Moregasm: Babeland's Guide to Mind-Blowing Sex*. In an article titled "How to Go Down on a Woman: Become a Cunnilingus Expert," she writes, "If it ain't broke, don't fix it. Most women orgasm in response to rhythmic stimulation, so if you're in a groove that is building her up, don't suddenly change what you're doing. Finding the balance between variety and consistency is the art to being an oral expert."[1]

Touch for Men

It doesn't take much to get most men excited, hence they don't always feel the need to linger in foreplay. They certainly don't have a problem teaching a woman how best to perform oral sex. The most important rule: no teeth. All manner of licking and stroking with your hands—in addition to using your mouth—will feel good to most men. If you are trying to make a baby, the goal in oral sex on men is to *not* bring him to orgasm, since you don't want to waste the sperm—it needs to head up into the vagina. Be sure to ask him what he likes—not as a topic of discussion, but during the act: "How does this feel? You like it? Guide me to where you'd like me to go."

Use your hands to play with your man's penis, or lingam as it is called in the Vedic tradition. Squeeze it, pull on it, push on it; be rough with it (but just don't try to bend it in half). Don't forget about the other erogenous zones men have, namely, the "family jewels" and the anus. Men love to have their testicles played with—gently, of course. The scrotal skin on top can be pulled and tugged but not so vigorously that you disturb the insides—that's where the sperm live. Another area men sometimes like to have stimulated is the anus—ask him if that's something he loves or would be willing to try. The best time to explore these erogenous zones is in the shower. There's something about the warmth of the water that feels so pleasurable. Using coconut oil, slather his whole body and then focus on the anal opening, home of thousands of nerve endings. If your man is into it, you can even gently slip your finger into his anus.

Sex Toy Shopping

Another sensual thing you can do is take a field trip for two to a sex toy shop. If you both feel a little sheepish about your outing—or afraid you might run into your neighbor or, worse yet, your boss—schedule it for an off-time. My partner and I decided to do just that one weekday morning, figuring no one goes to a sex shop on a Tuesday at 10 a.m. We chose The Pleasure Chest, a famous West Hollywood adult store that's been around since 1971. I walked around the store, trying to look as nonchalant as possible, and found myself in the party section. I picked up something called Weekend in Bed, described as a "kit for lovers." It included two adult card games as well as a paddle, a feather, a blindfold, a flogger, a candle, and, of course, a satin bag to put them all in. I moved on to the next aisle, where I found vibrators, dildos, and G-spot stimulators of all shapes, sizes, and colors. Just as I reached for an unusual-looking vibrator, a lanky young man with spikey red hair walked up and asked us if he could help. "Are you looking for anything in particular?" I went into "research" mode and replied, "I want to know how all these toys can help couples have more fun."

VIBRATORS: Most women are familiar with these toys (at least in theory), so it made sense to start there. Technology clearly had brought many more options than I thought possible. "Spike" told us that technology has given us myriad options, from USB-rechargeable sex toys with better, quieter motors, to ones that have a variety of speeds, shapes, and vibrations. As he held one up, he told me it not only vibrated, it thrusted as well. Not useful for fertility, I thought. I wanted to know more about clitoral stimulators, like the kind sex-toy expert, clinical sexologist, and certified sex coach Sonny Rogers told me about (Sonny is the resident sexual health educator for Pipedream Products, Jimmyjane, and Sir Richard's, all of which sell clitoral stimulators). When I asked her why she likes them so much, she told me the vibration from a stimulator "brings blood into the vulva, engorges the tissues, and helps get a woman wet and aroused." Her top four clitoral stimulators are listed below.

TOYS OF GLASS: Spike showed us an array of glass dildos in beautiful colors, kind of like the glass animal collection I had when I was in elementary school, only naughtier. They can heat up and are easy to clean, according to Spike. Sonny told me that dildos and life-size vibrators are more appropriate for same-sex couples. Many men don't like dildos, she says, "because they feel like they should be inside the woman instead."

FOUR SEX TOYS FOR WOMEN

Jimmyjane Form 2 by Jimmyjane

This clitoral stimulator, which looks like a set of rabbit ears, is powerful and flexible as well as waterproof and washable. Feel free to use it in the bath or shower. Named the #1 Sex Toy of the Year in 2009 by Fleshbot, Jimmyjane Form 2 has four vibration modes and five power levels.

Magic Wand by Hitachi

I love how this one is marketed as a personal massager—everyone knows what it's really used for! There are a lot of Magic Wand imposters out there, but this is the real deal. With its lower oscillation setting and deeper vibration than most massagers, women who have a harder time reaching orgasm love it. Sonny Rogers, the toy expert, advocates getting the regular Magic Wand, not the rechargeable one, because sometimes the power can go out in the middle of a precious moment, she says. Comes with plenty of cool attachments. And don't forget, it actually *can* be used to massage your partner's aching muscles.

Zumio

This toy is a bit like a sonic toothbrush on crack. It mimics the circular motion of a fingertip and vibrates superfast, which means it can cause a woman to reach orgasm fast, thanks to its SpiroTIP technology. Woman-designed, the Zumio won the 2017 Best New Product award at the Adultex, an adult trade show.

Womanizer

I must admit I don't love the name. But truth be told, there's nothing like it in the sex toy world. Created by a husband-and-wife team in Metten, Germany, this toy has a suction cup for the clitoris, and its technology makes it possible to stimulate the clitoris indirectly. It comes in different shapes, including one that looks like a lipstick for travel. Emily Morse, host of the podcast *Sex with Emily*, recommends it.

Toys for Men

Men can play, too—there are no shortage of toys for them. Spike showed us a sampling of what's available: prostate massagers, a.k.a. male G-spot stimulators, which come in different sizes and can go up a man's anus; anal plugs, which fit snugly into the anus while you're having intercourse; and a vibrating cock ring—one of Sonny's favorites—that gives both partners pleasure. The Pleasure Chest had a variety of cock rings—also called C-rings or penis rings—even disposable ones. The beauty of cock rings is that they can be applied when a man is semihard, making his erection last quite a bit longer because it keeps blood in the penis. It can be useful for a man who has difficulty maintaining an erection. You can gently put the cock ring on at the base of the penis, and include the balls; that is called a "fruit basket," or you can place it just at the base of the penis, without the balls. Don't leave a stretchy cock ring on for more than twenty minutes, however. Any of the basic cock rings made by Screaming O—Ringo, Screaming O Original Vibrating Ring, and Big O—will get you started.

Toys for Couples

There are a number of toys both partners can use during foreplay or intercourse to spice things up. We-Vibe, a clitoral and G-spot vibrator, is one. It takes some getting used to, but I hear once you do, it's enjoyable. Use it during intercourse and your partner will feel the vibe, too. Another one to check out is Eva, an egg-shaped vibrator that sits on top of the vulva and has wings that tuck into the labia. Women can use this hands-free while maintaining an intimate connection with their partner. Introducing stimulators like this doesn't mean that one partner is inadequate. Think of them as conversation-starters, a way of mixing things up.

Toys for Same-Sex Couples

I was pleased to see toys that simulate a penis, which same-sex couples can use to inseminate each other. One such device is called the POP (formerly known as the Semenette), which allows partners to mimic traditional intercourse and re-create the ejaculation process by using an inner tubing and pumping system. The mission of POP's creator, Stephanie Berman, was to provide an LGBTQ-friendly product to help same-sex couples conceive. She was pleased to report that POP does, in fact, work. She and her wife used it to conceive their daughter. She told me that with this device you can use either fresh or frozen sperm. Fresh is ideal for ICI (intracervical inseminations)—it's less expensive, and if you're using a known donor it's probably free. If you go the sperm-bank route, Stephanie suggests purchasing ICI-ready sperm and not IUI-ready (intrauterine) sperm because "insemination with the toy will only coat the cervix and not go directly into the uterus."

TAKING MATTERS INTO THEIR OWN HANDS

Bonnie and Leila had been together for a long time when they decided they wanted a baby. They both went to a fertility doctor to get checked out. "I never felt so old until they graded my eggs; I felt like a vagina-saur," said Leila. A close male friend of theirs agreed to be the donor. After trying IUIs that were costly and unsuccessful, they decided to take matters into their own hands. They invited their friend to their house, asked him to make a deposit in the next room, leave it at their bedroom door, and let himself out. They then used an oral syringe and inseminated each other, intracervically (ICI). Because their menstrual cycles were not in sync, they did this every two weeks for six months. They'd heard that having a sensual moment or orgasm would increase their chances, so they took advantage of that advice. "We managed to create orgasms to up our chances," Bonnie said. And the best part? "We laughed through the whole thing." They had great sex during that time. When I asked about foreplay, Leila said, "It's *all* foreplay! We used to use more tools, but we discovered that strap-ons are not sexy!"

Eventually, they went back to the fertility doctor and did IVF. They now have a beautiful girl, and their donor is a social figure in their child's life but not a legal parent. Although same-sex couples can't conceive the old-fashioned way, they can make their own baby-making journey connected and fun.

Sex toys are now a $15 billion industry. Couples who use them can often bring a lifeless sex life back to a sizzling one. Why not experiment with a few—just for fun? If you are going to use them, however, we need to have a conversation about lubrication—the kind to use on the toys themselves, as well as the cervical mucus women produce during their fertility window.

LUBRICATION

Do you know what cervical fluid is? Many of the women I treat haven't a clue. I never did either, not until I was attempting to get pregnant. My mother never told me about the wetness, the off-white fluid that would coat my panties. I was too embarrassed to ask what this moisture was, why it was there, and where it came from.

According to Dr. Christiane Northrup, author of *Women's Bodies, Women's Wisdom*, "women's vaginas have a cyclic sexual response of lubrication—about every fifteen minutes throughout the sleep cycle."[2] This lubrication makes it easier for the penis to glide into the vaginal opening and up near the cervix. So the more lubricated you are, the more you'll enjoy sexual penetration. However, lubrication isn't everything—don't equate wetness with readiness; think of it instead as the first step. A woman is wet *and* ready when her clitoris becomes engorged with blood and very sensitive, her vagina elongates, and the inner third of her vagina balloons out, lifting the uterus and cervix to receive an engorged and enlarged penis. This changed shape, along with a well-lubricated cervix, further facilitates the sperm-to-cervix journey.

Fertile cervical fluid has a property known as *spinnbarkeit*, "spinnability," which refers to the stringy or stretchy property found in vaginal mucus and to varying degrees in saliva at the time of or just prior to ovulation—probably between day twelve and fourteen of a twenty-eight-day menstrual cycle. It has the consistency of raw egg whites and is more alkaline than the sticky, creamy kind produced during the rest of the month. Note that sperm thrive in alkaline environs.

Some women produce very little fertile cervical mucus, and others none at all. Surgery on the cervix, infection from an STD, certain medications like antihistamines, allergy medications, or even the fertility drug Clomid are all possible culprits. Fortunately, there are herbs and nutritionals that can help the body make cervical fluid or thin it out. A supplement I sometimes recommend, besides herbs, is N-acetylcysteine, an antioxidant. Other practitioners prefer other nutritional supplements and herbs to balance the hormones. Check with your practitioner to figure out what's best for you. Being lubricated helps intercourse be more enjoyable.

Remember, if you need a little extra help, you can always reach for the lube. But when you're making a baby you can't choose just any lube.

What Not to Use

~ Stay away from synthetic lubricants. Most of them, like K-Y Jelly or Astroglide, contain petrochemicals that not only kill sperm, they can also harm or irritate vaginal flora. So that also means no Vaseline or baby oil either. As Wendy Strgar, founder of Good Clean Love, points out, some of these same petrochemicals can be found in brake fluid and antifreeze—definitely not an endorsement for putting them on your sensitive tissues.

~ Stay away from lubes that contain preservatives and other ingredients that may alter a woman's hormonal balance or create an imbalance of vaginal flora. Read the ingredient list on the packaging and steer clear of anything that lists parabens, including methyl-, ethyl-, and propylparabens, known estrogen disruptors; glycerin or glycerol, a byproduct of sugar that can irritate mucous membranes and sometimes make a vagina more prone to infections; propylene glycol, also used in antifreeze products; and chlorhexidine gluconate, which can cause irritation and inflammation.

~ Don't use lubes from the hospital because they often contain antiseptics that kill sperm, according to Dr. Paul Turek, who specializes in men's reproductive and sexual health.

What Works Best

~ Natural works best as far as I'm concerned. During ovulation, use a lube that has a pH of greater than 7, which provides the more alkaline environment that sperm can live in. YES Baby Pack 1 (from YES Baby) is sperm-friendly and organic. Another product approved by the FDA for fertility is Babydance by Fairhaven Health. This product doesn't contain parabens. During the rest of the month reach for lubes that have a more acidic pH of 4.4 or less, which is typical of the nonovulating vagina.

~ Raw egg whites work during ovulation, too, because they don't kill sperm (though I have trouble with the idea of sticking egg whites up my vagina).

~ Vegetable-based lubricants like olive oil, safflower, or coconut oil are all sperm-friendly, as Dr. Turek points out, and best for a woman's vaginal flora. Don't use the same bottle of oil you cook with; keep a separate one in your bedroom.

What about saliva as a lubricant? I asked Dr. Turek what he thought. "Not a good idea to use spit," he says. When men use spit to masturbate and then collect samples in fertility labs, the profusion of enzymes in saliva basically kill off all the sperm. He adds, "Enzymes that can digest meat can certainly digest sperm." Ugh. This really puts a damper on having oral sex, doesn't it? Most ob-gyns and reproductive endocrinologists agree that if you are going to go down on a woman, don't get slobbery; focus on the clitoris so that the saliva doesn't make it into the vagina and up in the cervix. Saliva is acidic, and the vagina needs an alkaline pH during the fertility window.

All of these pros and cons, back and forths about lubrication brings me right back to the most tried-and-true method of sending sperm on their baby-making journey: a woman's own cervical mucus. And the best way to make that happen? Plenty of foreplay! The whole point of foreplay is to enhance intimacy and connection. It's not always a prelude to sexual intercourse. If you are going through fertility treatments and sex is off the table, that doesn't mean you can't enjoy being sensual. It can be as simple as holding hands while taking a walk around the block, making each other a cup of tea and enjoying it together, or leaving each other love notes. With all the complications life has to offer, sometimes the best foreplay is to remember that your beloved is special and to treat them so.

SEXUAL SECRET
This tantra puja can get you both in the mood for love!

One of the best ways to get in the mood for baby-making love is to create a ritual around romance.

~ Create a sacred space for the two of you to come together (refer to chapter 10).
~ With devotion, honor your partner by offering her or him a special drink, singing a love song, or reciting a poem—either one you've written or one you've found that beautifully describes your feelings. Or get creative and design your own ritual.

These simple acts of love can create intimacy by melting away any obstacles that have accumulated during the day. If nothing else, it can enliven your playful nature—which would definitely be the case if I ever tried to sing a love song to my beloved!

15

The Big O

....

Only the united beat of sex and heart
together can create ecstasy.

—ANAÏS NIN

DO YOU REMEMBER THE SCENE in *When Harry Met Sally* when Sally shows Harry how women fake orgasms? The buildup, the moaning and crooning, eyes rolling back in ecstasy, and the grand finale were all so convincing that a woman sitting at a table nearby flagged a waiter down and said, "I'll have what she's having." Thinking back on that movie reminded me of my college years. I lived in a three-bedroom apartment with four other roommates, only one of whom had her own bedroom. She was having an affair with her professor and she would often invite him to spend the night in her room behind its very thin walls. Everyone could hear them going at it—she had rather vocal orgasms. We all agreed that we felt a little embarrassed and more than a little envious—okay, a little turned-on by it all, too. Who *doesn't* want what they're having? The fact is, experiencing it (even secondhand) is a lot more exciting than writing about it. But it's an essential topic, especially in a book as focused on creating intimacy and igniting passion as it is on baby-making. It's especially relevant because for many women, orgasms continue to be an elusive goal.

First, let's review. So far we've homed in on some key ways of bringing the deliciousness back into lovemaking. We've shown how seduction and foreplay are essential to "get the party started," so now's the time to bring everything to a climax. It's true, as many of my patients will admit, that women don't always have an orgasm even during regular lovemaking, and baby-making sex can make it almost impossible. They often ask me questions like, "I don't think I've ever had an orgasm. Is that a problem?" or even more specifically, "Do I need to have an orgasm in order to get pregnant?" No, it's not a problem; in fact, it's relatively common for women to not have an orgasm during sex. One journal article claimed that 50 percent of women don't orgasm through penetrative sex, and nearly 10 percent say they've never had an orgasm, even with self-pleasuring.[1] On the second question, let me reiterate and reassure you: you do *not* need to have an orgasm to make a baby.

Some women aren't sure if they've ever had an orgasm, so I think it's helpful right off the bat to define what an orgasm is. Most people agree that it's the pinnacle of sexual excitement, characterized by feelings of intense pleasure that can often pulsate throughout the whole body. For most men, orgasm and ejaculation appear to happen simultaneously, but they are different physiological responses to sexual pleasure. Technically, men can ejaculate without orgasm—a condition called *orgasmic anhedonia*; or they can orgasm without ejaculating. The former, as one man admitted, is not very enjoyable; it can be linked to depression, addiction, hormonal imbalance, or particular medications, and luckily it's quite rare. The latter is an antiaging practice that Taoists have long taught to help men not only live longer, but also have more pleasurable orgasms.

So why are we even talking about the "Big O" in a book about intimacy and fertility if we don't need one to make a baby? Three reasons: First, while they may not be necessary, orgasms may quite possibly get the semen moving more quickly in the right direction. Second, orgasms build trust, trigger a sense of euphoria, and can create a deeper bond with your beloved. And third, they're good for your health.

Get things moving. Orgasms "draw ejaculated semen into the uterus," according to Barry Komisaruk, a psychology professor at Rutgers University and the co-author of *The Orgasm Answer Guide*.[2] This is what's called the "up-suck" theory and it goes something like this: When a woman has an orgasm during sex, her pituitary gland releases the "cuddle hormone," oxytocin, which causes the uterus to contract quite forcefully, multiple times. The suction created by these wavelike contractions, Komisaruk says, is what draws semen up and deposits it near the cervix. The theory goes that a woman who has an orgasm after the man has ejaculated into her (or, for lesbian couples who use a syringe to conceive, right after sperm is inserted) will suction the sperm up as a result of orgasmic contractions.

Pamela Madsen, author of *Shameless: How I Ditched the Diet, Got Naked, Found True Pleasure . . . and Somehow Got Home in Time to Cook Dinner* and a popular sexuality, pleasure, and relationship consultant, wrote an article for *Psychology Today* titled "What Does Sex Have to Do with Fertility?" In it, she says that women have a "magic ring of engorgeable tissue" that fills with blood whenever "your body surrenders to pleasure." This ring of pleasure "helps the sperm stay closer to the entrance of the uterus," she writes, "which is where we want it to be." She goes on to explain that when these special tissues engorge with blood, "the 'round ligaments' of the uterus contract," which allows the cervix to move toward the back of the vaginal canal—an invitation to the sperm to move "right into the opening of the cervix and into the uterus, to eventually meet with your waiting egg."[3]

Build deeper trust. The ability to orgasm is inexorably tied to our ability to trust and to surrender in the moment. To forget that you're ovulating, to relax into simply being pleasured and giving pleasure, with no agenda, no thought of trying to control the outcome—that is what's required for conception, even when you time intercourse perfectly (via the natural route or with Western reproductive medicine). Orgasm goes beyond just climaxing; it's a whole-body experience, an exquisite release that engenders a sense of euphoria and a deeper bond with your partner. Orgasm is like an energy dance, a pulsating drive to connect, followed by a sweet release. Nicole Daedone, author of *Slow Sex*, says, "Orgasm fundamentally roots our capacity for connection: hormonally, emotionally and spiritually."[4]

Benefit your health. Besides getting the sperm moving, orgasms offer some pretty amazing benefits—more reasons to get busy! They can lower blood pressure, increase circulation, reduce premenstrual and headache pain (without decreasing sensitivity), help you sleep better, and, studies suggest, even look younger.[5] Women report that more frequent lovemaking keeps their genital tissues healthy and supple—the "use it or lose it" theory.

The inside scoop. When we get sexually excited, DHEA increases; oxytocin, the "love hormone," surges just before orgasm, perhaps accompanied by a flood of endorphins, those natural pain relievers; and the brain releases dopamine, another feel-good neurotransmitter, during ejaculation in men and orgasm in women. One study suggests that the neurohormone prolactin increases with sexual satisfaction.[6] And oxytocin continues to stay elevated after we're lovingly nestled in each other's arms. It's important to understand, however, that most of these benefits come more from making love, less so from self-pleasuring. For example, the prolactin increase following intercourse for both sexes is 400 percent greater than that following masturbation.[7] Prolactin is also one of the hormones—along with oxytocin—responsible for your mate falling asleep after sex. Now I understand why my husband could never stay awake after we made love, no matter how much I nudged!

WHAT PREVENTS ORGASM?

Before listing all the reasons a woman doesn't have an orgasm, I just want to reiterate: don't worry if you're not. Good sex promotes good health, but good sex doesn't always mean having a rocking, body-shaking orgasm. Oxytocin is released through hugging, kissing, genital stimulation—anything that makes a woman feel desired, aroused, and connected. And this rise in oxytocin decreases the stress response, orgasm or no orgasm. So don't discount giving and receiving pleasure with no other goal in mind.

Now then, why don't more women have orgasms? What gets in their way? Truth be told, many women don't even know if they have or they haven't. Everyone wants the "happy ending," but not everyone knows how to make that happen. Women have confided in me that they often fake orgasm, which I discovered was not at all unusual. Relationship and sex therapist Patricia Futia did a study on orgasm and mindfulness for her dissertation, in which she interviewed a hundred women ranging in age from twenty to over sixty. She found that 90 percent had faked orgasm at least once. And the number-one reason they gave? They weren't enjoying the sex act and wanted it to end. The number-two reason was that they wanted to assuage their partner's ego.[8] Studies show (no surprise) that a man judges himself harshly if he can't bring his partner to orgasm. The third reason was they want to be thought of as multiorgasmic and a great lover.

In addition to these reasons, there are several others that can account for why couples can't make that happy ending happen:

Unresolved emotions: The inability to share difficult emotions that often arises when the goal of having a baby seems impossible— resentment, anger, fear, sadness, anxiety—can make it difficult for couples to be intimate. As well, negative past experiences that resulted in distrust or shame or trauma can definitely prevent women from letting go and being vulnerable.

Stress: For many couples, nothing is more stressful than trying (and failing) to get pregnant. With the added pressures to eat just the right foods and to make love (or withhold love) at exactly the right time, plus wondering why and how and what conspired to keep them childless, who has the time or the desire to create a loving, sensual, satisfying scene in the bedroom? Some couples opt for assisted medical reproduction to ease the male partner's burden of having to ejaculate on demand.

Weak pelvic floor: According to Michael Castleman, a journalist who has written about sex research for more than thirty-five years, when the muscles in the pelvic floor, which contribute to ejaculation and orgasm, are weakened, "semen doesn't spurt, it dribbles, and orgasms may provide little pleasure."[9]

Giving without receiving: Castleman calls this the "delivery boy attitude": when a man focuses all his attention on giving pleasure, he "loses erotic focus, which can interfere with ejaculation and orgasm."[10] That can happen to women, too, of course—especially when their partner is less interested in sensual foreplay and more interested in getting the job done.

Drugs: Myriad drugs can interfere with the body's ability to climax. Blood pressure meds, alcohol, marijuana, pain relievers, antianxiety and antidepression drugs—especially SSRIs (selective serotonin reuptake inhibitors)—are particularly troublesome for couples trying to conceive. Reading the common side effects of these drugs, says Catherine Pearson, in her article "This Is Your Orgasm on Antidepressants," is like "flipping through a grim catalog of potential sexual dysfunction. Decreased sex drive. Decreased sexual performance. Men can experience impotence. Women can lose feeling in their vaginas and nipples. Studies have shown that both sexes can experience diminished and delayed orgasms, or none at all."[11] Unfortunately, doctors are often all too eager to prescribe SSRIs for someone suffering from anxiety and depression, without taking into consideration the fact that he or she is trying to make a baby. Many of my patients say they've been able to get to the heart of their depression by trying things like herbal and nutritional supplements, acupuncture, body-based trauma-sensitive therapy, hypnosis, yoga, and an array of other mindfulness modalities. Of course, if you are already on antianxiety or depression meds, never, ever go off of them without a doctor's supervision.

Bad technique: A woman might not know what she needs to climax or where it comes from (no pun intended). Clitoral stimulation may get her off when she does it herself, but not when she and her partner make love. What gives? It could be that her partner doesn't know how to stimulate her to orgasm. Maybe the pressure is too much or not enough; maybe her partner doesn't hit the right spot or spend enough time on her clitoris. And no doubt she has trouble admitting that her lover isn't satisfying her. Communicating about sexual needs is difficult. Don't give up, though. With the right stimulation and practice, orgasm *can* happen.

TYPES OF ORGASMS

The jury is still out on how many and what kinds of orgasms women are capable of having. Many agree with sex therapist Ian Kerner, author of *She Comes First: The Thinking Man's Guide to Pleasuring a Woman*, who believes that *all* orgasms are clitoral and they're too often dismissed as "being quick and lighthearted, while the others are somehow deemed more serious and substantial."[12] Even if a woman comes during vaginal penetration, he says, chances are she's having a clitoral response. Others say sexual release is much more complicated than that. In her book *Orgasms for Two*, artist and feminist sexologist Betty Dodson, PhD, gives us what she believes is the winning orgasm combo: a blend of clitoral stimulation, vaginal stimulation, PC muscle contractions, pelvic thrusting, and breathing out loud. During intercourse, the woman or her partner simply adds her preferred kind of clitoral contact. Studies confirm Dodson's observation. According to a 2018 study published in the *Archives of Sexual Behavior*, "women were more likely to orgasm if their last sexual encounter included deep kissing, manual genital stimulation and/or oral sex, in additional to vaginal intercourse."[13]

With all that in mind, here are a variety of orgasm types to ponder and perhaps to try:

Clitoral Orgasm

One of my patients declared with absolute conviction that if her husband "would just attend to my clitoris for a while, I probably would come. But he doesn't spend enough time down there." She's certainly not alone. In a 2017 internet survey conducted with women age eighteen to ninety-four, the majority said clitoral stimulation was the key to "erotic satisfaction," while 37 percent said clitoral stimulation was essential, and another 36 percent said it vastly improved their orgasms.[14] According to Castleman, "Over my 40+ years as a sexuality journalist and counselor, I've heard many psychologists insist that women's sexuality is so complicated and individual that the 'cookbook' advice found in 'sex manuals' is simplistic and largely beside the point. Perhaps. But with all due respect to women's emotional complexity, this study [a 2015 study of partner satisfaction] shows that the key to women's erotic satisfaction and orgasm is the sex itself, specifically direct clitoral stimulation."[15]

G-Spot Orgasm

Sex and relationship coach and self-described "vaginal weightlifter" Kim Amami believes any woman can have this orgasm. Unlike the clitoral orgasm, however, which she says is mostly physical, the G-spot requires a woman to be emotionally ready; she must feel safe, open, and vulnerable. Find the G-spot, which is on the anterior (front) wall of the vagina—it's a rough or rigid patch that you stimulate with a come-hither motion. Some women like pressure on it, others prefer that it be rubbed in a circular motion. Some women climax quickly with G-spot stimulation, while others take as long as thirty minutes. Because the Skene's glands are near the G-spot, a woman can ejaculate or release a fluid sometimes called amrita or "sweet nectar." Taoists say absorbing a woman's jing secretions gives long life to men.

Women can activate their own G-spot and learn how to ejaculate or "squirt," but don't expect to squirt like a fire hose like they do in porn.

AFE (Anterior Fornix Erogenous) Zone, a.k.a. the A-Spot Orgasm

This area of sensitivity is located at the deepest point of the vagina, on the upper (anterior) wall, where it begins to curve upward above the G-spot.

The Deep Spot Orgasm (Posterior Fornix Orgasm)

This is the posterior (toward the back) part of vaginal wall near the cervix. This area can be stimulated by the penis if penetration is made by rear entry.

U-Spot Orgasm

This happens by stimulating the tissue around the urethral opening.

Cervical Orgasm

Some women like their partner to give their cervix a little love, others don't. Some say it feels too much like having a pap smear.

Breast Orgasm

Massaging the breasts, especially around the nipples, can bring some women to orgasm. Combining breast play—pulling, sucking, tugging, biting the nipples—with clitoral play can enhance orgasm.

Whole-Body Orgasm

Nothing is quite as amazing as a whole-body orgasm, and sexologists say it's available to any woman willing to open herself up emotionally and physically. This tantra-inspired orgasm often begins with clitoral or penile stimulation. As you become excited, you begin to focus on moving the sexual energy up from the lower chakras to the upper ones, using a combination of full breaths, moans and groans, and a squeezing and releasing motion of the pelvic muscles (think Kegels). Whole-body orgasms can happen without clitoral or penile stimulation, too, by pumping the PC muscle to move the energy up the spine. You can do this by yourself or with a partner, intercourse optional. (As well, refer to the chakra breathing exercise in chapter 4.)

Eco-Spot Orgasm

Ecosexuality, a term coined by X-rated feminist, former porn star, and "ecosexual" Annie Sprinkle and her partner, Beth Stephens, is at the intersection of sexuality and ecology. That's the rather dry, scientific definition for what is a juicy invitation. Ecosexuals take Earth as their lover; they seek to feel a deep, intimate, sensual connection with all that is nature—often to the extent that they can have an orgasm just being in a meadow or forest or garden. To ecosexuals, Earth is not necessarily feminine, but

Annie Sprinkle doesn't care what pronoun you use, she just wants you to find your E-spot, that place on Earth that turns you on. She wants you to feel so in love with nature that you will never harm anything.

Sex Magic

Sounds like voodoo perhaps, but why not, at the moment of orgasm, set an intention to invite in the spirit of your unborn child? Some say this practice is from ancient times and is included in some tantra teachings. Use the power of this creative and magnificent orgasmic energy to manifest and co-create a child. At the very moment of orgasm, look into each other's eyes and declare, either silently or out loud, "We are making a baby!"

Multiple Orgasms

Women are capable of having multiple orgasms—approximately 47 percent of them do, according to statistics posted on the educational research website OMGYES. Some women experience them in rapid succession, others require a pause before going again. A friend of mine confessed that his girlfriend needs him to remain still and not move for about ten minutes before she can climax again. So yes, we know that women can have multiple orgasms, but what about men? Sex researchers William Hartman and Marilyn Fithian, authors of *Any Man Can: The Revolutionary New Multiple Orgasmic Technique for Every Loving Man*, investigated the male multiple orgasm and defined it as two or more orgasms without losing an erection. And why do we care? Most women would laugh at that question—of course we care, because multiple orgasms bring more pleasure and extend lovemaking time. Western medicine weighs in by saying that it's important for men to ejaculate in order to keep the prostate healthy. Of course, baby-making orgasms should ultimately end in ejaculation so that the sperm can get moving and find its egg mate.

Taoist master Mantak Chia, author of *The Multi-Orgasmic Man: Sexual Secrets Every Man Should Know*, says, "In the East, the Taoists have long known that orgasm could be a whole-body experience and developed techniques for expanding orgasmic pleasure. . . . With practice, you can learn to experience the peak feeling of orgasm without triggering the reflex of ejaculation."[16] That's all well and good, however, climaxing without ejaculation isn't helpful when you're trying to make a baby. Sometimes men do find their energy flags after ejaculating. That can indicate low Kidney energy according to Chinese medicine. When that happens, it's time to fortify with kidney tonic herbs and conserve your jing by not ejaculating too much during the nonfertile weeks.

TOO MUCH, TOO SOON: Some men don't have any problem ejaculating—they just jump the gun and do it prematurely. It's not necessarily worrisome for couples because the sperm do make their way into the vagina; however, in this case a woman doesn't have enough time to have her own orgasm and up-suck the sperm (and doesn't enjoy herself nearly as much as she'd like). Premature ejaculation can happen for myriad reasons, such as stress, performance anxiety, depression, and injuries; it can also be a side effect of medication. Some men just learned to do it fast and need to learn a new style (see chapter 5 for an array of techniques). Betty Dodson suggests changing position may delay ejaculation and even give women more time to have an orgasm. Other strategies include using numbing creams that contain lidocaine or experimenting with a cock ring (see chapter 14). Sometimes antidepression meds such as SSRIs can help men suffering from depression-related performance issues, although reproductive urologist Philip Werthman doesn't recommend them for men trying to get their partner pregnant because these meds have been shown to increase sperm DNA fragmentation—in other words, they're not good for sperm.

What Can Couples Do?

First of all, stop worrying and stop asking. When you take the pressure off trying to reach orgasm and focus on pleasurable sensations for both of you instead, sex can be much more fulfilling. Women claim it's a big turnoff to be constantly asked "Are you close?" "Did you come?" Instead, just feel into the moment and make your move.

GO IT ALONE AT FIRST: Betty Dodson and others in the field of sexology recommend that women learn how to orgasm through self-pleasuring.

As Dodson says, "Sex is a skill that we learn; it doesn't come naturally like people think." She often suggests that women begin by discovering what's up down there (see chapter 1) and then, using a vibrator, center on clitoral stimulation and pleasure. When women know what turns them on, they can teach their partners what to do.

TAKE THINGS SLOW: You can learn how to have an orgasm as a couple by not focusing on intercourse at all for a while. Think of a whole night of just being touched on different parts of your body—the nape of your neck, your inner thigh, lips, ears, fingers, and toes—and moaning in ecstasy. Picture every cell's inner battery being charged and your whole body lighting up, giving off a golden glow that awakens the senses. Don't be surprised if you climax—but don't think of that as a goal. Just enjoy mutual pleasure.

MIX THINGS UP: Women are complicated. What works for us on Tuesday might not work on Thursday. If you can't find your sweet spot, experiment with pressure, timing, rhythm. That said, don't give up on something that's a sure thing. A patient of mine wondered if her sexual habits were normal. "We probably only have sex twice a week, is that okay?" she asked. "My husband comes pretty quickly, but then he finishes me off after so I have an orgasm."

"Does that work for you?" I asked her. "Do you feel satisfied?"

"Yeah, it's great!"

There's your answer: "if it's ain't broke, don't fix it!"

DON'T STOP TOO SOON: When Betty Dodson coaches women on how to achieve an orgasm, she'll often blurt out, "Stay in it!" when she sees them giving up just when orgasm is right around the corner. Charles Muir, founder of the Source School of Tantra Yoga, says that women will often short-circuit their sexual energy when they get close to orgasm because they forget to breathe.

DON'T BE AFRAID TO ASK FOR WHAT YOU WANT: You may be unable to achieve an orgasm because your partner needs a little help in the sex department. Or your styles and timing are just different enough that neither of you feels satisfied. One of my patients told me that it took her a while to tell her husband that she needed something in her vagina during oral sex—like his finger or a sex toy—in order to climax. One day she found a blog post about that very thing. She sent it to him and . . . he got it! Problem solved.

BE HONEST WITH EACH OTHER–ABOUT EVERYTHING: Sometimes what prevents us from true sexual pleasure is everything else that's happening in our lives. If something bugs you about your partner and it prevents you from feeling connected and loving, put it on the table and discuss, if you can. Don't be afraid to seek help to facilitate those conversations. My patient Lee is a prime example. She frequently felt like there was a something stuck in her throat that prevented her from speaking. In Chinese medicine, we refer to this as stuck throat energy or "plum-pit qi." She couldn't tell her partner that she was worried about their finances and wished he would take a more active role in saving money. She couldn't tell her partner that she had suffered from bulimia in her twenties, was still having episodes, and was afraid that would affect her fertility. She couldn't tell her partner what she needed in order to orgasm. She benefited from acupuncture treatments, Chinese herbal medicine, and therapy. Once her throat chakra opened up, she was able to be more honest, and as a result their relationship became more intimate.

LET THE WOMAN TAKE THE LEAD while the man pays attention to her energy and to signs—or for same-sex couples, choose which one to lead. Synchronize your breathing; ride her wave and wait for her to reach orgasm first—either with oral or manual stimulation. In *Art of the Bedchamber: The Sexual Yoga Classics Including Women's Solo Meditations* translated by Douglas Wile, a man must look for signs that the woman is experiencing pleasure. When her desire for orgasm reaches the greatest intensity, Taoists say, her body will go straight and her eyes will close.

BRING A SENSE OF ORGASM INTO YOUR LIFE: Regardless of how you reach orgasm during lovemaking—or if you ever do—what's really important is that you infuse your life with pleasure and purpose—in and out of the bedroom. Orgasm is a state of mind, a way of approaching life's challenges and joys with determination, clarity, and wholehearted enthusiasm. Having said that, don't give up the quest for orgasmic sex.

Play, experiment with different positions, talk to each other in ways that encourage exploration, or even redefine what orgasm means for you both—without being attached to the outcome. Seek not only a fulfilling sex life, but a fulfilling relationship and a fulfilling life.

SEXUAL SECRET
Learn the Taoist method of intensifying orgasm.

Tn *The Sexual Teachings of the White Tigress: Secrets of the Female Taoist Masters*, Hsi Lai, a contemporary Taoist teacher, introduced the West to a three-thousand-year-old tradition in which women learned sexual and spiritual practices to increase their beauty and realize their feminine nature. Admittedly, this ancient tradition addressed courtesans, but still, the author's understanding of men and women and their sexual energies is useful. Hsi Lai says that a woman's sexual energy descends: it begins in her mouth, flows to her breasts, and lands in her vagina. These are called the "Three Peaks." Following this order can increase a woman's sexual secretions. A male's energy, on the other hand, ascends, starting with the penis. Think of the yin/yang symbol. The black portion on the right represents female energy (yin) in its full expression moving downward, while the white portion on the left represents male energy (yang) and points upward.

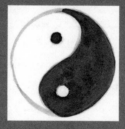

16

When You Need a Hand

....

There's a crack, a crack in everything
That's how the light gets in

–LEONARD COHEN

THIS SECTION FOCUSES ON what most couples never talk about at a dinner party (even though we've all witnessed some cringe-worthy exceptions): what happens when you've done everything right and you still haven't been able to conceive? Most of us would have difficulty talking to a close friend about it, let alone announcing to our book club that our husband has trouble performing. Face it, it's damn hard to bare your perceived inadequacies or share your concerns without a lot of embarrassment or shame.

But honestly, don't be afraid to seek help if you need it, before giving up. I've had patients who admit they turned to Western reproductive medicine too quickly because it was easier than dealing with their sexual issues. Hal Danzer, MD, a reproductive endocrinology and infertility specialist and the co-founder of the Southern California Reproductive Center, finds it interesting that couples don't talk to him that much about sex, even though "sexual dysfunction is so common," he says. That doesn't leave couples with a lot of places to turn to process their feelings. It's important to have a support team, a few people you can trust; it helps you put things in perspective when you feel like you're losing it or when you feel like nothing is ever going to get better. Even the Yellow Emperor, who ruled

China from 2697 to 2598 B.C., had three female sexual advisors—the Plain Girl, the Harvest Girl, and the Mystery Girl—and one male doctor. The most famous of these advisors was the Plain Girl, known as Su-Nu. The emperor's questions on sexuality were recorded in *The Plain Girl's Classic* (Su-Nu Ching) between the third and fourth century B.C. How else was he going to find out how to keep up with his many concubines?

SHY PENIS SYNDROME

This is a common concern, albeit an embarrassing one. There are myriad reasons why some men can't get it up, keep it up, or empty it out. Let's take a look at some of the causes, and then we'll offer a few remedies.

For the record, the scientific name for shy penis syndrome is erectile dysfunction, or ED, although I personally love the term "yang wilt," from traditional Chinese medicine. The kind of ED we're talking about here is called secondary or situational ED, which means it's caused by something else; primary ED is when you've never been able to maintain an erection.

Causes

Erections are all about blood flow, and when the blood isn't flowing, the penis isn't responding. "Some men have blood-flow issues, plain and simple," says Kathryn Retzler, MD, in an interview she did with Mike Mitzel for the podcast *High Intensity Health*. "In men over forty, 80 percent of ED is caused by microplaque."[1] That's a fancy name for clogged veins in the penis. The first thing a urologist will rule out is cardiovascular disease (who says the heart and penis aren't connected?). Other culprits include high blood pressure and other medical conditions, certain medications, smoking, low testosterone, relationship issues, stress, trauma, and depression.

Performance and IVF

With the calendar dictating the timing of everything, the pressure to get it up can be too much, and the poor penis wilts before it ever makes it to the grand finale, the victory orgasm. One husband whose wife was in the throes of IVF told me how embarrassing—and near impossible—it was for him to leave his deposit at the clinic. "You should have seen the man who came out of the room before I went in. He had to carry his specimen through the waiting room and ask the nurse where to put it. He couldn't even look up. When it was my turn, it was hell. I turned on the TV, all the porn I could watch was right there. But I'm not even into porn these days. And it was ten o'clock in the morning—not exactly my optimal time."

Solutions

For any physiological concerns, the first thing is to get checked out by a reproductive urologist to make sure nothing's clogged. If low testosterone is the problem, don't supplement. Taking additional testosterone, doctors say, fools your body into thinking it has enough so that the testicles don't have to make any—which in turn will cause your testicles to shrink and sperm counts to be severely reduced.

I know it's going to sound strange coming from a natural-solutions acupuncturist, but if medications, stress, or even relationship issues prevent you from getting and sustaining an erection, you might want to consider a little pharmaceutical assistance. Just to make sure, I asked reproductive endocrinologist and infertility specialist, Richard Marrs what he advises when one of his patients has difficulty making his sperm deposit. He said he definitely offers the Viagra option. If you don't want to pop the blue pill in the bedroom you could try a pump or a cock ring—available at adult pleasure stores or online—both of which force blood into the penis, which helps you sustain an erection.

Caution: Get some help if you want to use one of these. The penis is a delicate appendage; you don't want to overpump it and cause problems.

NITRIC OXIDE: Increase your intake of foods and supplements that increase production of nitric oxide. This chemical compound, which the body manufactures, relaxes arterial walls, dilates blood vessels, and improves the flow of blood—all of which can help with brainpower (the big brain) and erections (the little brain). Supplements such as citrulline, L-arginine, grape seed extract, pycnogenol, and CoQ_{10} can increase nitric oxide production. Foods that will increase it include beets and arugula, as well as fresh spinach, citrus, walnuts, and watermelon (which contains high levels of citrulline).

ACUPUNCTURE AND TRADITIONAL CHINESE MEDICINE TREATMENTS: Obviously, while Viagra and Cialis are fine to get the party started, it's important to get to the root of the problem. In other words, we want to treat the whole tree, not just one branch.

LOW-INTENSITY SOUND WAVES: There's a device called a Gainswave (go.gainswave.com), which uses low-intensity sound waves to break up microplaque in the penis. It purports to increase nitric oxide production and improve collateral blood flow within four to twelve weeks, according to Dr. Retzler.

QIGONG: If you want your erections to last longer, be stronger, and more sensitive, make sure you're healthy. Taoists call this "preparing for clouds and rain" (clouds being vaginal secretions, rain being semen), says Kenneth S. Cohen in his book *The Way of Qigong*. Besides this solution, you can practice the Male Deer exercise, described in this chapter, to help you address shy penis syndrome and enhance your overall fertility and sexuality.

A CAUTIONARY TALE

A couple came to see me. She was thirty-two and he was thirty-five. They both wanted a baby but they knew that they had to get healthy first. He had been a prizefighter, had overdosed on recreational drugs, and had developed heart arrhythmia. He confessed that he had taken steroids for a long time because they made him feel like the Hulk. But that was before he had an up-close-and-personal brush with death—and that had freaked him out. But what he really wanted to talk about was his "other" problem—his cock. It had stopped working. I told him I wasn't surprised; his problem no doubt stemmed from his use of anabolic steroids, which interrupt the body's ability to produce testosterone on its own. The result? Low sex drive and depression. First thing to do was to restore the body's yang energy. To do that, I put him on an adrenal yang tonic. I also wrote him a formula to increase blood flow around his heart, which had become enlarged. Because in Chinese medicine the heart and the reproductive organs are energetically linked, blood flow to the heart would help alleviate his erectile problems. He recovered, albeit slowly, and was thrilled when his penis began to work again.

THE MALE DEER EXERCISE

This is best practiced in the morning, naked below the waist, and, if possible, with an erection.

1. Sit on a chair or cross-legged on a pillow; take a few gentle, deep breaths to relax your body and get present.
2. Cup the right hand around the testicles gently and rest the right thumb on the base of the shaft of the penis.
3. With the left hand, massage the area between the navel and pubic bone, called the *dantian*, in a clockwise motion eighty-one times.
4. Repeat with the opposite hand.
5. Place your hands on your lap and rest for several breaths. Your hands should be in fists, with the thumbs enclosed.
6. Now contract the perineum muscles (between the tailbone and the genitals) without tensing any other muscles—especially in your shoulders, face, and jaw; breathe normally. Work up to one minute and then relax completely for one minute. Repeat this step nine times.

PAINFUL SEX

If sex is painful for you, you're definitely not alone—anywhere from 10 to 20 percent of women in the United States suffer from vaginal pain.[2] Painful intercourse is called *dyspareunia*; chronic pain affecting the vulva and opening of the vagina is called *vulvodynia*, *vestibulodynia*, or *vulvar vestibulitis* syndrome. If you experience either problem, make an appointment with your ob-gyn to figure out what's going on.

Causes of Dyspareunia

STRESS: Overthinking, inability to relax, the pressure of having to make a baby—all of this conspires to make lubrication a challenge and sex quite literally a pain. Sometimes the solution is as simple as relaxation techniques and more foreplay.

TRAUMA OR SEXUAL ABUSE: Unprocessed emotions or buried memories of childhood or adult sexual abuse can surface during this time.

MEDICAL CONDITIONS: Endometriosis, cysts, fibroids, infections (even after they've been cleared up), pelvic-floor dysfunction, side effects of certain medications, and skin conditions can all cause pain.

HARSH PRODUCTS: Irritating soaps, detergents, and lubricants can cause irritation to tissues. Be sure to use only chemical-free and fragrance-free products (with organic ingredients as much as possible). Check out the lube information in chapter 14.

PELVIC-FLOOR ISSUES: Most women haven't a clue what's going on with their pelvic floor and wouldn't know if it's too tight, too loose, or too weak. But as physical therapist Dustienne Miller says, "When people have pain, they can have any combination of tightness and weakness in the pelvic floor." Deena Poll Goodman, a physical therapist and women's health specialist, says there could be "trigger points, tight muscles, or nerve issues that are affecting the muscles, causing tissue irritation and pain."

Causes of Vulvodynia

The cause of vulvodynia is less understood. According to Andrea Rapkin, director of the UCLA Chronic Pelvic Pain and Vulvodynia Program, this condition can occur because of any number of factors: hormonal changes; inflammation; pelvic-floor problems; irritation from soaps, detergents, and panty liners; or even changes in brain processing or a disruption in pain signals for the vaginal area.

Solutions

If you are experiencing any kind of pelvic pain, make an appointment with your ob-gyn to rule out anything unusual. There are plenty of experts who focus on pelvic pain, such as medical doctors, pelvic-floor physical therapists, somatic bodyworkers, sex therapists, acupuncturists, herbalists, and psychotherapists. The decision to make a baby can bring up issues long buried or forgotten, and the journey to heal your genitals can provide freedom to the individual and the couple.

PHYSICAL THERAPY: Deena Poll Goodman also says there are "so many variables when it comes to pelvic pain, so it's important to seek health-care professionals who specialize." She says PT works well for dyspareunia (painful sex), vaginismus (spasms of the vaginal muscles when something enters), and anorgasmia (when the inability to orgasm causes personal distress). Deena herself draws on manual therapy, visceral mobilization, cold laser, ultrasound, electrical stimulation, and therapeutic exercise, including mind-body integration patterns, to help her clients. A pelvic pain specialist will generally do muscle testing vaginally and rectally, Goodman says, to assess both movement and strength. If a patient is in a lot of pain, she may opt to do an external assessment of the muscles instead so she doesn't cause more pain or create more tension.

If you are having pelvic pain, check out videos from Dustienne Miller, who integrates yoga with pelvic-floor exercises. You can find her at Yourpaceyoga.com.

INTEGRATIVE APPROACHES: The therapeutic program at UCLA's Chronic Pelvic Pain and Vulvodynia Program uses medications, topical hormones, diet, acupuncture, yoga, mindfulness-based meditation, and cognitive-behavioral therapy, as well as specific muscle treatments; addresses the neuropathic components of pain; and prescribes surgery if it is warranted.

CHINESE MEDICINE: Traditional Chinese herbs and acupuncture can help to decrease pain and inflammation. It's particularly effective for women who have endometriosis, fibroids, painful menstruation, pelvic inflammatory disease, PMS, irregular bleeding, and vulvodynia.

O-SHOTS AND P-SHOTS: A colleague of mine, Robyn Benson, a doctor of Oriental medicine and owner of the clinic Santa Fe Soul, gives O-shots and P-shots, based on the work of Charles Runels, MD. These shots contain platelet-rich plasma (PRP) spun from your own blood and are injected into your female or male parts. Sounds painful, I know, but Robyn insists it doesn't hurt. Women who have sexual arousal disorder, orgasmic disorder or pain, and bladder problems may benefit from this treatment. For men, she says, the P-shots helps with erectile dysfunction. This might be worth looking into (see the resources section at the end of the book).

MISCARRIAGE OR EARLY TERMINATION

No words can describe the pain couples feel when they miscarry or when their baby dies in utero. The grief is unbearable, and the subsequent fear and worry that arise when they decide to try again seem insurmountable. Lucretia and Benjie were one of those couples. Lucretia was in her forties, and after not having much luck with her own eggs, decided to go the donor-egg route. She was one of the healthiest women I've ever worked with, and her pregnancy was worry-free. She exercised, ate well, and gained just the right amount of weight. She positively glowed. Everything changed the day she went into her doctor's office at thirty-six weeks pregnant. The baby wasn't moving and the doctor couldn't find a heartbeat. The baby had died of a cord accident, and Lucretia was forced to deliver the baby vaginally. Her phone call broke my heart. Her grief was inconceivable. She saw a counselor, joined a grief support group, and tried to reimagine her life. Losing a child is like that. What could I possibly say to her? All I could do was offer love and treatments that would support her process. I suggested doing a ceremony to celebrate the life of her baby girl. She and Benjie went down to the beach and tossed white roses into the ocean.

A year passed before they were ready to try again. It would be an understatement to say that they were concerned during the pregnancy. But with support from Benjie and her extended family and friends, weekly acupuncture and lots of prayers, Lucretia birthed a healthy baby girl. "She really is a little miracle," Lucretia said. "It was hard, but it's so important to keep moving forward in life. I can say I'm truly blessed, and I'm not one to say that type of thing."

Suggestions

CREATE A CEREMONY: Ritual has the power to heal. I often suggest that couples plant a tree in honor of their lost child, toss flowers into a running stream or the ocean, or write a letter or poem to their baby. One of my patients took her partner to a lantern festival where thousands of lanterns were let go into the night sky. As she sent hers skyward, she felt that she had symbolically let go of her loss in order to slowly move forward.

JOIN A SUPPORT GROUP: While there are plenty of support groups for those who are grieving, you may find it beneficial to seek out those specifically for women (or couples) who have lost children to miscarriage or had a late-term intrauterine fetal death.

BE PATIENT AND KIND TO YOURSELF: There is no right way to grieve and there's no timetable for how long to grieve. You will no doubt always feel the loss—and that is perfectly normal. Remember that the intense fluctuation of hormones that happens postmiscarriage will also ensure that the body-mind-heart balance will take more time than you imagine.

GET CHECKED OUT BY YOUR PHYSICIAN: You should always see a physician after a miscarriage to make sure everything has been expelled. If you've had recurrent pregnancy losses—two or more miscarriages—you'll want the doctor to look for what may have caused them.

ACUPUNCTURE AND CHINESE MEDICINE: I've helped many women and men heal from miscarriage so they can begin to try again. When working with acupuncture and grief, we place the needles in such a way that they can access the energy in the body where the qi has become stuck. These emotional, spiritual, and physical blockages put us in direct contact with the wisdom of the body so that the healing process can begin. Acupuncture and herbal medicine can also help rebalance hormones and rebuild the body.

PRACTICE GRATITUDE: One way to do this is by practicing the Inner Smile meditation found in chapter 13. Direct your gratitude first to your reproductive organs, thanking them for the work they do, and then thank all of your organs and glands.

FIND A SOMATIC HEALER: Sometimes a miscarriage can trigger other traumatic experiences that have become embedded in your cells. Talk therapy doesn't always work because as discussed in chapter 11, unprocessed emotions live in the body and must be dislodged. Kimberly Ann Johnson, a sexological bodyworker, Somatic Experiencing practitioner, yoga instructor, and the author of The Fourth Trimester, says that women can benefit from somatic healing even before they go to their gynecologist postmiscarriage, especially if they've been triggered. Through touch and somatic practices, Johnson gives women the experience of what it's like to listen to their bodies so that they can heal the wounds of the loss they carry within.

WHEN CAN YOU TRY AGAIN?

Paul Crane, MD, has been an ob-gyn for more than thirty years, although he may be best known for giving Kim Kardashian a sonogram on TV. When I asked him when couples could try to get pregnant again after a miscarriage, this was his reply: "I'd like couples to wait one normal cycle, because some evidence suggests that if a woman gets pregnant before that, there could be a higher risk of a second miscarriage."

Second Time Around

Most couples who already have a child never even consider that they'd have trouble the second or third time around. So when that happens, it can really send them into a tailspin. Suddenly, all they can think about is *What if we never have another child? What if one of us is suddenly infertile? But how could that be? We've already had a child! Maybe my eggs dried up. Maybe we're too old. Maybe, maybe, maybe . . .* In the meantime, of course, they're missing out on the life they're nurturing already. Myriad possibilities account for this second fertility challenge, not the least of which may be the added stress of being parents *and* wage earners, which cuts into the time and energy they used to have for lovemaking. It could even be that they can't quite believe they're capable of conceiving again or they feel guilty for wanting more than what they already have.

My patient Marci is a good example. She really wanted a second child—all her friends had at least two and a few were on their third. Because she got pregnant easily the first time, she thought it would be a piece of cake the second time around. It didn't happen that way. After trying for months, they opted for IVF—and that didn't work either. By the time Marci walked into my clinic, defeated and sad, she and her husband weren't even having sex anymore. She had completely forgotten that her body was capable of conceiving, capable of experiencing pleasure. All she knew was that it had betrayed her. What was my advice?

NURTURE YOURSELF: Take time to reestablish your physical, emotional, and mental vitality, which has no doubt dimmed in the process of trying to do it all—be a mom, work, get pregnant. Start by attending to your own womb space and rekindling your goddess self. Self-care is key. Eat nourishing foods, exercise, get a massage—anything that recharges your energy. And then get back to self-pleasuring to awaken your mojo.

NURTURE YOUR RELATIONSHIP: As Marci discovered, her obsession with having another child left little room for anything else, especially her relationship with her husband. They never had a night off to themselves, and sex was limited to procreation as dictated by a fertility calendar. Changing diapers and breastfeeding were hardly conducive to feeling desirable or aroused, but with a little creativity—and friends who babysit—Marci says they've been able to slowly get back to making love for fun and pleasure, and not just to make babies.

BABY-MAKING POSITIONS: TRUE OR FALSE?

The jury's still out. In fact, there's really no research to suggest one position over another—only many theories. And yet women trying to conceive are forever trying to stay on their backs with a pillow under their butt because they've read that's how to get sperm closer to the cervix. And we definitely want to get sperm as close to the cervix as possible. For many, that means the missionary position or even doggie-style. But it really all depends on the position of your uterus. The missionary-style (man on top) works for any woman who has a normally positioned uterus. But as Paul Crane explained to me, for someone who has a retroverted uterus—a uterus that's tilted backward, about 20 percent of all women—it doesn't work as well as doggie-style, i.e., the man entering the vagina from the rear.

Anna Davies, who wrote "Best Sex Positions to Conceive a Baby" for bump.com, says the reverse cowgirl is a position better suited to a woman with a retroverted uterus. I hadn't the foggiest idea what that meant. Did it have something to do with riding a horse or milking a cow? I looked it up. It's a position in which the woman is on top and faces away from a man's face. It doesn't work for everyone—as one of my patients said, "I'm not an acrobat in Cirque du Soleil"—so you might be more comfortable sticking with doggie-style.

Should we really be limiting how we have sex to the best position for making a baby? I say no! Honestly, don't add more have-tos to your list. Mix things up; just make sure the position makes you sufficiently aroused. Books like the Kama Sutra have all kinds of crazy positions to try, with names like "Magic Mountain" and "The Mermaid." One website (www. babymed.com/love/kama-sutra-sex-position) has descriptions of a hundred positions. And of course, there's always *The Joy of Sex*, the classic book on positions written in 1972 by the aptly named Alex Comfort.

The truth is, when a woman is juicy and her cervix is open, those sperm travel fast. Dr. Crane says that having good, fertile cervical mucus "will catch some of the sperm right away," so you can even make love standing up if you wish. If you're worried that too much sperm is going to fall out in this position, Dr. Crane says put a pillow under your butt for ten to fifteen minutes afterward to hold everything in. Regardless of whether one position works better than another, commit to a little aftercare and spend time together bonding in the glow of your connection. It might be just the encouragement the sperm needs to swim to their destination.

SEXUAL SECRET
It's All about Love

Here is the best-kept secret of all: It's all about LOVE. As Mahatma Gandhi says so eloquently, "Where there's Love, there's Life." So, don't be in such a rush to get to the finish line that you allow the flame of your passion to flicker and die. You are creating life out of the love you have for each other. Savor every moment—the joys *and* the disappointments, the laughter and the tears—because it's all part of the journey. Use what you've learned in this book to help you rediscover a sense of intimacy, reignite your passion, and become a sexual adventurer!

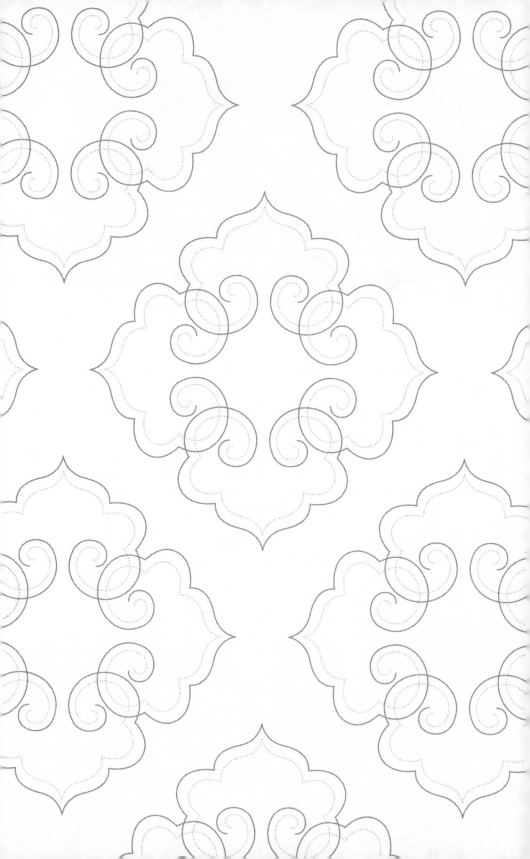

Acknowledgments

A big thank you:

To Linda Sparrowe: You are an incredible light. Without you I couldn't ever have accomplished such a project. You made it easy to write about sex. To Steve Adams, for putting me in touch with the right person at the right time and telling me my book would be evergreen. Because of you this book is a reality.

To my editor at Shambhala, Beth Frankl, thank you for believing in this book and how it will help women and men! To my copy editor, Margaret Jones, proofreader, Ashley Benning, and associate editor, Audra Figgins, thank you for your valuable input. To my amazing illustrator, Wren Polansky, you are an artist and so wonderful to work with. To Katy Seeger, thank you for taking time to help me be a visionary.

To my children Noah and Ethan who had to deal with sex books all around the house as I researched—you are both a blessing!

To my mother, Annette Tucker, a songwriter herself, thank you for believing I had a talent for writing. To my father, Morey Wiesner, you love with your big heart. And to Adam Sheck, for your support while I wrote and talked endlessly about the book. Thank you for your love, passion, and patience.

To my mentors:

Randine Lewis: Knowing you, learning from you, and being friends with you has changed my life. Amara Charles: You are the definition of what it means to be a healer and have helped me understand sexuality. Sheyna: You have showed me what it means to fully embrace your femininity and your sexuality. Patti Britton: Thank you for creating Sex Coach University and for being the warm caring person you are. Thank you to my writing teacher Jack Grapes who encouraged us all to wear the hat.

Thank you to the remarkable practitioners of the Fertile Soul and ABORM. I learn from all of you every day.

To Trudy Goodman and Jack Kornfield: Your relationship and teachings are grounded in love. You both live the dharma.

To Barry Komisaruk: I was honored to have your brilliant research mind help me with one of my chapters. To all the amazing MDs that gave me their time and openly shared with me their impressive knowledge: Dr. Hal Danzer, Dr. Carolyn Alexander, Dr. Catherine DeUgarte, Dr. Richard Marrs, Dr. Andy Huang, Dr. Eric Surrey, Dr. Paul Magarelli, Dr. Paul Turek, Dr. Philip Werthman, and Dr. Paul Crane. Patients are lucky to be in your care.

Thank you to all the gifted healers and practitioners that graciously shared their wisdom and expertise. You are all impressive: Kia Miller, Dustienne Miller, Deena Goodman, Sheri Winston, Betty Martin, Jessica Durivage, Laura Catone, Hala Khori, Uma Dinsmore-Tuli, Dr. Hyla Cass, Heather Askinosie, Hazel Williams-Carter, Ray Sahelian, Sunny Rogers, Dan Holman, Wendy Strgar, Sarah Brooke, Jani White, Melanie Alexander, Dr. Patricia Futia, Niika Quistgard, Peter Holmes, David Emerson, Robyn Benson, Dr. Emily Morse, Sarah Marshank, Celina Criss, Zoë Kors, Sari Cooper, Kimberly Ann Johnson, Lori Snyder, Dawn Cartwright, Helen Adrienne, Kathryn Simmons-Flynn, Barbara Harper, Robyn Goldberg, Linda De Villars, Yaron Seidman, Dean Sluyter, Rodika Tchi, Niraj, Kiki Lovelace, Jayme Barrett, Brenda Strong, Jai Uttal, Heather Rhea Dawn, Dr. Kim Bergman, and Eden Fromberg.

To all the people who supported me to make this book possible: Alan, Dale, Gloria, Lisa, Laura, Michael, and Chase.

To my esteemed colleagues and staff at Natural Healing & Acupuncture: Teresa, Katya, Emily, Anna, Jolee, and all others: You are like family.

And to all of my fertility patients: You are my teachers. Thank you.

Notes

CHAPTER 1. WHAT'S UP DOWN THERE?

1. Catherine Pearson, "Lets Clear Up the Vagina vs. Vulva Debate Once and for All." *Huffington Post*, Oct. 28, 2015. Available online.
2. Priscilla Frank, "Artist's Unapologetic Vagina Paintings Are a Force of Body Positivity." *Huffington Post*, Feb. 21, 2017. Available online.
3. Leslie Rickey, "Straight Talk about Sex and the Pelvic Floor with Leslie Rickey, MD," www.pericoach.com.
4. A. L. Pastore, "Pelvic floor muscle rehabilitation for patients with lifelong premature ejaculation: A novel therapeutic approach." *Therapeutic Advances in Urology* 6, no. 3 (2014): 83–88.
5. Amara Charles interviewed by author Jan. 9, 2016. See also Amara Charles, *The Sexual Practices of Quodoushka: Teachings from the Nagual Tradition*. Rochester, Vt.: Destiny Books, 2011.
6. Jolan Chang, *The Tao of Love and Sex*. New York: Penguin, 1977, p. 84.

CHAPTER 2. WET AND HARD

1. A. R. Hirsch and J. J. Gruss, "Human male sexual response to olfactory stimuli." *American Academy of Neurological and Orthopaedic Surgeons* 19 (1999): 9–12.
2. A. L. Cerda-Molina, L. Hernández-López, C. E. de la O, R. Chavira-Ramírez, and R. Mondragón-Ceballos, "Changes in men's salivary testosterone and cortisol levels and in sexual desire after smelling female axillary and vulvar scents." *Frontiers in Endocrinology* 4 (2013): 159.
3. S. Kuukasjärvi, C. J. P. Eriksson, E. Koskela, T. Mappes, K. Nissinen, and M. J. Rantala, "Attractiveness of women's body odors over the menstrual cycle: The role of oral contraceptives and receiver sex." *Behavioral Ecology* 15, no. 4 (2004): 579–84.
4. Carla Clark, "Brain Sex in Men and Women from Arousal to Orgasm," www.brainblogger.com, May 20, 2014.
5. C. J. Charnetski and F. X. Brennan, "Sexual frequency and salivary immunoglobulin A (IgA)." *Psychological Reports* 94, no. 3, pt. 1 (2004): 839–44.
6. Sari Cooper interviewed by author July 27, 2017.
7. Rosemary Basson, "Rethinking low sexual desire in women," *BJOG* 109, no. 4 (2003): 357–63.
8. Pamela Madsen, "The Arousal Principle: The Complexity and Simplicity of Female Erotic Desire." *Huffington Post*, March 9, 2015. Available online.
9. M. L. Chivers, G. Rieger, E. Latty, and J. M. Bailey, "A sex difference in the specificity

of sexual arousal." *Psychological Science* 15, no 11 (2004): 736–44. "This helps explain why medications such as Viagra have a significant effect for men, but don't really do much to help a woman's sexual desire (even though it does the same thing physically for women as it does for men—helps their erectile tissue fill with blood)."

10. Madeleine Castellanos, "Differences for Sex Start in the Brain," www.thesexmd.com.

11. Katherine Wu, "Love, Actually: The Science behind Lust, Attraction and Companionship." Harvard University *Science in the News*, Feb. 14, 2017. Available online.

12. A. Aron, E. Melinat, E. N. Aron, R. Vallone, and R. Bator, "The experimental generation of interpersonal closeness: A procedure and some preliminary findings." *Personality and Social Psychology Bulletin* 23 (1997): 363–77.

13. R. Munarriz, N. N. Kim, I. Goldstein, and A. M. Traish, "Biology of female sexual function." *Urologic Clinics of North America* 29, no. 3 (2002): 685–93.

14. David Levine, "Anthropologist and Love Expert Helen Fisher on the Mysteries of Love: An Interview with the Chief Scientific Advisor for Match.com—and the brains behind the Chemistry.com personality test." *Elsevier*, July 29, 2014. Available online.

CHAPTER 3. THE RISE AND FALL OF PASSION

1. "New Survey Finds Infertility Delivers a Serious Blow to Self-Esteem." *Cision PR Web*, Sept. 15, 2018. The survey of 585 women and men was conducted in September 2009 by GfK Roper on behalf of Schering-Plough. Article available online.

2. Helen Adrienne interviewed by author July 3, 2016.

3. T. H. Chen, S. P. Chang, C. F. Tsai, and K. D. Juang, "Prevalence of depressive and anxiety disorders in an assisted reproductive technique clinic." *Human Reproduction* 19, no. 12 (2004): 2313–18.

4. A. Babore, L. Stuppia, C. Trumello, C. Candelori, and I. Antonucci, "Male factor infertility and lack of openness about infertility as risk factors for depressive symptoms in males undergoing assisted reproductive technology treatment in Italy." *Fertility and Sterility* 107, no. 4 (2017): 1041–47.

5. D. Hooper, A. Tenforde, and A. Hackney, "Treating exercise-associated low testosterone and its related symptoms." *Physician and Sports Medicine*, Aug. 27, 2018.

6. D. Vaamonde, C. Algar-Santacruz, A. Abbasi, and J. García-Manso, "Sperm DNA fragmentation as a result of ultra-endurance exercise training in male athletes." *Andrologia* 50, no. 1 (2018).

7. Joe Dispenza, *Breaking the Habit of Being Yourself: How to Lose Your Mind and Create a New One.* Hay House, 2012, pp. 22, 25, 59.

8. Stan Tatkin, *Wired for Love: How Understanding Your Partner's Brain and Attachment Style Can Help You Defuse Conflict and Build a Secure Relationship.* Oakland, Ca.: New Harbinger Publications, 2011, p. 17.

9. Adam Sheck interviewed by author Feb. 7, 2017.

CHAPTER 4. PLEASURE TRADITIONS FROM THE EAST

1. Jane Lyttleton, *Treatment of Infertility with Chinese Medicine*. London: Churchill Livingstone, 2004, p. 12.
2. R. Yehda, N. P. Daskalakis, L. M. Bierer, H. N. Bader, T. Klengel, F. Holsboer, and E. B. Binder, "Holocaust exposure induced intergenerational effects on FKBP5 methylation." *Biological Psychology* 80, no. 5 (2018): 372–80.
3. Giovanni Maciocia, "Shen and Hun: The Psyche in Chinese Medicine," Nov. 30, 2012. Available online.
4. Lonnie S. Jarrett, *The Clinical Practice of Chinese Medicine*. Spirit Path Press, 2006, p. 8.

CHAPTER 5. THE ART OF SELF-PLEASURING

1. G. Giorgi and M. Siccardi, "Ultrasonographic observation of a female fetus' sexual behavior in utero." *American Journal of Obstetrics and Gynecology* 175, no. 3, pt. 1 (1996): 753.
2. R. Fernández and R. López, "In utero gratification behaviour in male fetus." *Prenatal Diagnosis* 36, no. 10 (2016): 985–86.
3. SIECUS, "Sexuality Information and Education Council of the United States," https://siecus.org/wp-content/uploads/2018/07/Position-Statements-2018-2.pdf.
4. Patti Britton, YouTube lecture based on Britton's *The Art of Sex Coaching: Expanding Your Practice*. New York: W. W. Norton, 2005.
5. "Sexual Health for the Millennium: A Declaration and Technical Document," www.worldsexology.org.
6. Noam Shpancer, "The Masturbation Gap: The Pained History of Self-Pleasure." *Psychology Today*, Sept. 29, 2010. Available online.
7. International Society for Sexual Medicine, "What is 'Edging' and Why It Might Be Employed," www.issm.info/sexual-health-qa/what-is-edging-and-why-might-it-be-employed.
8. Anna Breslaw, "Why All Men Should Be Edging during Sex." *Cosmopolitan*, May 6, 2014. Available online.
9. Philip Werthman interviewed by author April 25, 2017.
10. M. A. Perelman, "Psychosexual therapy or delayed ejaculation based on the Sexual Tipping Point model." *Translational Andrology and Urology* 5, no. 4 (2016): 563–75.
11. Leon F. Seltzer, "What Distinguishes Erotica from Pornography." *Psychology Today*, April 6, 2011. Available online.
12. Naomi Wolf, *Vagina: A New Biography*. New York: HarperCollins, 2012, p. 249.
13. Marty Klein, *His Porn, Her Pain: Confronting America's PornPanic with Honest Talk about Sex*. Santa Barbara, Ca.: Prager, 2016, pp. 112–13.

CHAPTER 6. TIMING IS EVERYTHING

1. S. A. Robertson, "Seminal fluid and fertility in women." *Fertility and Sterility* 106, no. 3 (2016): 511–19.

2. J. R. Kovac, R. P. Smith, M. Cajipe, D. J. Lamb, and L. I. Lipshultz, "Men with a complete absence of normal sperm morphology exhibit high rates of success without assisted reproduction." *Asian Journal of Andrology* 19, no. 1 (2017): 39–42.

3. Paul Turek interviewed by author Feb. 28, 2018.

4. Philip Werthman interviewed by author April 25, 2017.

5. Paul Magarelli interviewed by author March 15, 2018.

CHAPTER 7. FINE-TUNING THE ENGINE

1. Gabrielle Roth, *Maps to Ecstasy: The Healing Power of Movement*, rev. ed. Novato, Ca.: Nataraj Publishing, 1998, pp. 29, 31.

2. Emily Bartlett and Laura Erlich, *Feed Your Fertility: Your Guide to Cultivating a Healthy Pregnancy with Chinese Medicine, Real Food, and Holistic Living.* Fair Winds Press, 2015, p. 25.

3. Linda De Villers, *Simple Sexy Food: 101 Tasty Aphrodisiac Recipes and Sensual Tips to Stir Your Libido and Feed Your Love.* Marina Del Rey, Ca.: Aphrodite Media, p. 27.

4. D. M. A. B. Dissanayake, P. S. Wijesinghe, W. D. Ratnasooriya, and S. Wimalasena, "Effects of zinc supplementation on sexual behavior of male rats." *Journal of Human Reproductive Sciences* 2, no. 2 (2009): 57–61.

5. S. Akarsu, F. Gode, A. Z. Isik, Z. G. Dikmen, and M. A. Tekindal, "The association between coenzyme Q10 concentrations in follicular fluid with embryo morphokinetics and pregnancy rate in assisted reproductive techniques." *Journal of Assisted Reproduction and Genetics* 34, no. 5 (2017): 599–605.

6. T. D. Gundersen, N. Jorgensen, A. M. Andersson, A. K. Bang, L. Nordkap, N. E. Skakkebæk, L. Priskorn, A. Juul, and T. K. Jensen, "Association between use of marijuana and male reproductive hormones and semen quality: A study among 1,215 healthy Young Men," *American Journal of Epidemiology* 182, no. 6 (2015): 473–81.

7. Mayo Clinic, "Erectile Dysfunction," www.mayoclinic.org.

8. "Couples' pre-pregnancy caffeine consumption linked to miscarriage risk." National Institute of Health news release, March 24, 2016 (available online); and G. M. B. Louis, K. J. Sapra, E. F. Schisterman, C. D. Lynch, J. M. Maisog, K. L. Grantz, and R. Sundaram, "Lifestyle and pregnancy loss in a contemporary cohort of women recruited before conception: LIFE Study." *Fertility and Sterility* 106, no 1 (2016): 180–88.

9. A. K. Chandrasekhar, J. Kapoor, and S. Anishetty, "A prospective, randomized, double-blind, placebo-controlled study of safety and efficacy of a high-concentration full-spectrum extract of ashwagandha root in reducing stress and anxiety in adults." *Indian Journal of Psychological Medicine* 34, no. 3 (2012): 255–62.

10. J. Waynberg and S. Brewers, "Effects of Herbal vX on libido and sexual activity in premenopausal and postmenopausal women." *Advances in Therapy* 17, no. 5 (2000): 255–62.

11. Yaron Seidman interviewed by author Aug. 1, 2017.

12. Laurie Mintz, *A Tired Woman's Guide to Passionate Sex: Reclaim Your Desire and Reignite Your Relationship.* Avon, Mass.: Adams Media, 2009, p. 19.

13. S. Fernando and L. Rombauts, "Melatonin: shedding light on infertility? A review of the recent literature." *Journal of Ovarian Research* 7 (2014): 98.

14. O. Hakimi and L. C. Cameron, "Effect of exercise on ovulation: A systematic review." *Sports Medicine* 47, no. 8 (2017): 1555–67.

15. A. C. Hackney, A. R Lane, J. Register-Mihalik, and C. B. O'Leary, "Endurance exercise training and male sexual libido." *Medicine and Science in Sports and Exercise* 49, no. 7 (2017): 1383–88.

16. B. Hajizadeh Maleki and B. Tartibian, "Moderate aerobic exercise training for improving reproductive function in infertile patients: A randomized controlled trial." *Cytokine* 92 (2017): 55–67.

CHAPTER 9. FIRE AND FLAME

1. Patricia Futia interviewed by author Nov. 20, 2017.

2. Lorie Eve Dechar, *Five Spirits: Alchemical Acupuncture for Psychological and Spiritual Healing.* New York: Lantern Books, 2006, pp. 173, 175.

3. K. Floyd, J. P. Boren, A. F. Hannawa, C. Hesse, B. McEwan, and A. E. Veksler, "Kissing in marital and cohabitating relationships: Effects on blood lipids, stress, and relationship satisfaction." *Western Journal of Communication* 73, no. 2 (2009): 113–33.

4. Dean Sluyter, *Natural Meditation: A Guide to Effortless Meditation Practice.* New York: Jeremy P. Tarcher/Penguin, 2015, p. 221.

CHAPTER 10. SETTING THE STAGE

1. Marie Kondo, *The Life-Changing Magic of Tidying Up: The Japanese Art of Decluttering and Organizing.* Berkeley, Ca.: Ten Speed Press, 2014, p. 178.

2. S. A. Mortazavi, S. Taeb, S. M. Mortazavi, S. Zarei, M. Haghani, P. Habibzadeh, and M. B. Shojaei-Fard, "The fundamental reasons why laptop computers should not be used on your lap." *Journal of Biomedical Physics and Engineering* 6, no. 4 (2016): 279–84.

3. N. N. Takasu and T. J. Nakamura, "Recovery from age-related infertility under environmental light-dark cycles adjusted to the intrinsic circadian period." *Cell Reports* 12, no. 9 (2015): 1407–13.

4. Jayme Barrett, *Feng Shui Your Life.* New York: Sterling Publishing, 2003, p. 182.

5. Jayme Barrett interviewed by author Nov. 9, 2017.

6. Heather Askinosie interviewed by author Sept. 18, 2017.

7. Heather Askinosie.

8. Met Museum, "Fertility Figure: Female (Akua Ba)," www.metmuseum.org/toah/works-of-art/1979.206.75/.

CHAPTER 11. HEALING TRAUMA, LETTING GO OF SHAME

1. Lonnie S. Jarrett, *The Clinical Practice of Chinese Medicine*. Spirit Path Press, 2006, p. 8.
2. Bruce Lipton, *The Biology of Belief: Unleashing the Power of Consciousness, Matter, and Miracles*. Hay House, 2005, p. 300.
3. Pro Seminars, "Ray Rubio: Why I Created the ABORM," www.prodseminars.net/story/ray-rubio-why-i-created-aborm.
4. Brene Brown, *The Gift of Imperfection: Let Go of Who You Think You're Supposed to Be and Embrace Who You Are*. Center City, Minn.: Hazeldon, 2010.
5. International Society for Sexual Medicine, "What Does 'Sex Positive' Mean?" www.issm.info/sexual-health-qa/what-does-sex-positive-mean.

CHAPTER 12. RELEASING STRESS

1. C. D. Lynch, R. Sundaram, J. M. Maisog, A. M. Sweeney, and G. M. B. Louis, "Preconception stress increases the risk of infertility: Results from a couple-based prospective cohort study—the LIFE study." *Human Reproduction* 29, no. 5 (2014): 1067–75.
2. K. Kircanski, M. D. Lieberman, and M. G. Craske, "Feelings into words: Contributions of language to exposure therapy." *Psychological Science* 23, no. 10 (2012): 1086–91.
3. B. G. Kalyani, G. Venkatasubramanian, R. Arasappa, N. P. Rao, S. V. Kalmady, R. V. Behere, H. Rao, M. K. Vasudev, and B. N. Gangadhar, "Neurohemodynamic correlates of 'OM' chanting: A pilot functional magnetic resonance imaging study." *International Journal of Yoga* 4, no. 1 (2011): 3–6.
4. Solala Towler, *The Tao of Intimacy and Ecstasy: Realizing the Promise of Spiritual Union*. Boulder, Co.: Sounds True, 2014.

CHAPTER 13. DEEPENING INTIMACY

1. Margo Anand, *The Art of Sexual Ecstasy: The Path of Sacred Sexuality for Western Lovers*. New York: Jeremy P. Tarcher/Putnam, 1989, p. 66.
2. Andrea Miller, *Radical Acceptance: The Secret to Happy, Lasting Love*. New York: Atria Books, 2017.
3. Gary Chapman, *The 5 Love Languages: The Secret to Love That Lasts*. Chicago, Ill.: Northfield Publishing, 2014, p. 35.
4. Celina Criss interviewed by author Sept. 25, 2017.

CHAPTER 14. FOREPLAY

1. Rachel Venning, www.babeland.com/sexinfo/mens-room/how-to-go-down-on-a-woman.
2. Christiane Northrup, *Women's Bodies, Women's Wisdom: Creating Physical and Emotional Health and Healing*. New York: Bantam, 1994, rev. ed., 2006, p. 238.

CHAPTER 15. THE BIG O

1. D. L. Rowland, L. M. Cempel, and A. R. Tempel, "Women's attributions regarding why they have difficulty reaching orgasm." *Journal of Sex and Marital Therapy*, Jan. 3, 2018: 1–10.

2. Barry R. Komisaruk, Beverly Whipple, Sara Nasserzadeh, and Carlos Beyer-Flores, *The Orgasm Answer Guide*. Baltimore, Md.: The John Hopkins University Press, 2010.

3. Pamela Madsen, "What Does Sex Have to Do with Fertility?" *Psychology Today*, June 7, 2013. Available online.

4. Nicole Daedone, *Orgasm: The Cure for Hunger in the Western Woman*, YouTube video for TEDxSF, www.youtube.com/watch?v=s9QVq0EM6g4.

5. "Top Ten Health Benefits of Orgasm for Women," www.floliving.com/top-10-health-benefits-of-orgasm-for-women.

6. S. Brody and T. H. C. Kruger, "The post-orgasmic prolactin increase following intercourse is greater than following masturbation and suggests greater satiety." *Biological Psychology* 71, no. 3 (2006): 312–15.

7. S. Brody and T. H. C. Kruger.

8. Patricia Futia interviewed by author Nov. 20, 2017.

9. "Many men have difficulty with ejaculation and orgasm." Michael Castleman, "Men's Secret Sex Problem," *Psychology Today*, March 15, 2012. Available online.

10. Michael Castleman.

11. Catherine Pearson, "This Is Your Orgasm on Antidepressants," *Huffington Post*, Feb. 16, 2016. Available online.

12. Ian Kerner, *She Comes First: The Thinking Man's Guide to Pleasuring a Woman*. New York: HarperCollins, 2004, p. 464.

13. D. A. Frederick, H. K. S. John, J. R. Garcia, and E. A. Lloyd. "Difference in orgasm frequency among gay, lesbian, bisexual, and heterosexual men and women in a U.S. national sample." *Archives of Sexual Behavior* 47, no. 1 (2018): 273–88.

14. D. Herbenick, T. J. Fu, J. Arter, S. A. Sanders, and B. Dodge, "Women's experiences with genital touching, sexual pleasure, and orgasm: Results from a U.S. probability sample of women ages 18 to 94." *Journal of Sex and Marital Therapy* 44, no. 2 (2018): 201–12.

15. "Trouble with orgasm? Personal history matters less than direct clitoral caresses." Michael Castleman, "Why So Many Women Don't Have Orgasms," *Psychology Today*, Feb. 1, 2016. Available online.

16. Mantak Chia and Douglas Abrams Arava, *The Multi-Orgasmic Man: Sexual Secrets Every Man Should Know*. New York: HarperCollins, 1996.

CHAPTER 16. WHEN YOU NEED A HAND

1. Kathryn Retzler, *GAINSwave & P-Shot for ED, Sexual Performance*, YouTube video for *High Intensity Health*, www.youtube.com/watch?v=8Hln5IVr5lA.

2. D. A. Seehusen, D. C. Baird, and D. V. Bode, "Dyspareunia in women." *American Family Physician* 90, no. 7 (2014): 465–70.

Resources

This section includes publishing information for sources mentioned in the book, cites additional resources and references, and is organized according to chapter and topics within those chapters.

CHAPTER 1. WHAT'S UP DOWN THERE?

Acupuncture. The American Board of Reproductive Medicine (ABORM) lists ABORM-certified practitioners (as well as information on how to become certified) on its website, www.ABORM.org.

Sexual practices. Amara Charles, *The Sexual Practices of Quodoushka: Teachings from the Nagual Tradition*, Rochester, Vt.: Destiny Books, 2011; Alain Danielou, trans., *The Complete Kama Sutra: The First Unabridged Modern Translation of the Classic Indian Text*, Rochester, Vt.: Park Street Press, 1994; and Nick Karras, *Petals*, San Diego, Ca.: Crystal River Publishing, 2017.

CHAPTER 2. WET AND HARD

Essential oils. Try Snow Lotus, created by Peter Holmes, L.Ac, MH, which are fully bioactive, artisan-quality essential oils: www.snowlotus.org. For breast massage oil, try www.livinglibations.com.

Sex, physiological aspects. "What Happens in the Brain during Orgasm," www.health.howstuffworks.com/sexual-health/sexuality/brain-during-orgasm1.htm; and "Your Brain on an Orgasm," www.womenshealthmag.com/sex-and-love/orgasm-body.

Sexual practice. Margo Anand, *The Art of Sexual Ecstasy*, New York: Jeremy P. Tarcher, 1989 (see pp. 78–82 on the whole-body/melting hug); Randine Lewis, *The Way of the Fertile Soul: Ten Ancient Chinese Secrets to Tap into a Woman's Creative Potential*, New York: Atria Books, 2007; and Mantak Chia and Michael Winn, *Taoist Secrets of Love: Cultivating Male Sexual Energy*, Santa Fe, N.M.: Aurora Press, 1884.

CHAPTER 3. THE RISE AND FALL OF PASSION

Counseling and therapy. Helen Adrienne, *On Fertile Ground: Healing Infertility*, Create Space, 2011; and for infertility counseling, mind-body therapy, and clinical hypnotherapy, see www.helenadrienne.com. Eva Clay, MSW, clinical sexologist, helps couples have deep, passionate, authentic sexual pleasure. www.evaclay.com. Adam Sheck, PsyD, www.thepassiondoctor.com.

Women's mysteries. Greta Hassel, licensed marriage and family therapist and sex educator, leads Red Tent Los Angeles, which hosts monthly gatherings of women that are filled with ritual and storytelling in celebration of women's mysteries—see www.redtentlosangeles.com.

CHAPTER 4. PLEASURE TRADITIONS FROM THE EAST

The Cock Project. Dr. Hazel Grace Yates offers an innovative, fun, and educational style of sex and intimacy coaching at www.drhazelgraceyates.com.

Universal Healing Tao. Master Mantak Chia teaches Taoist sexual cultivation at his Universal Healing Tao website, www.universal-tao.com.

CHAPTER 5. THE ART OF SELF-PLEASURING

Education. International Society for Sexual Medicine, www.issm.info; Planned Parenthood, www.plannedparenthood.org; Sexual Information and Education Council of the United States (SEICUS), www.siecus.org; Source School of Tantra Yoga, www.sourcetantra.com; and the World Association for Sexual Health (WAS), www.worldsexology.org.

Masturbation and sex play. For information on the Betty Dodson method of self-love and feminist-based sex education, including masturbation videos, go to www.dodsonandross.com; see also Lou Paget, *How to Be a Great Lover Girlfriend-to-Girlfriend: Totally Explicit Techniques that Will Blow His Mind*, New York: Random House, 1999.

Ovarian breathing and Taoist microcosmic orbit breathing. Mantak Chia, *Healing Love through the Tao: Cultivating Female Sexual Energy*, Rochester, Vt.: Destiny Books, 2005.

Porn. Marty Klein, *His Porn, Her Pain: Confronting America's Porn Panic with Honest Talk about Sex*, Santa Barbara, Ca.: Praeger, 2016.

CHAPTER 6. TIMING IS EVERYTHING

Fertility clinics and reproductive urology clinics. California Fertility Partners, Dr. Richard Marrs and associates, www.californiafertilitypartners.com; CMD Fertility, Dr. Catherine DeUgarte. www.cmdfertility.com; Center for Male Reproductive Medicine and Vasectomy Reversal (CMRM), Dr. Philip Werthman, www.malereproduction.com; Colorado Center for Reproductive Medicine (CCRM), Dr. Eric Surrey, www.ccrmivf.com; Growing Generations, the first surrogacy and egg donation agency devoted to serving the gay and lesbian community, www.growinggenerations.com; HQA Fertility Centers, Dr. Paul Magarelli, www.hqafertilitycenters.com; Huntington Reproductive Centers (HRC), Dr. David Tourgeman, Dr. Diana Chavkin, and associates, www.havingbabies.com; Reproductive Partners, Dr. Andy Huang and associates, www.reproductivepartners.com; Southern California Reproductive Center (SCRC), Dr. Hal Danzer, Dr. Carolyn Alexander, and associates, www.scrcivf.com; and The Turek Clinics, Dr. Paul Turek, www.theturekclinic.com.

Fertility self-help. Jani White, *The Fertile Fizz*, Strandweaver Press, 2016; World Health Organization (WHO) guidelines for sperm and Kruger strict criteria, www.who.int/reproductivehealth/topics/infertility/cooper_et_al_hru.pdf; and for a quick reference guide to semen analysis, www.fertilityauthority.com/story/semen-analysis-quick-reference-guide.

CHAPTER 7. FINE-TUNING THE ENGINE

Acupuncture/acupressure. Deborah Bleecher, *Acupuncture Points Handbook: A Patient's Guide to the Locations and Functions of over 400 Acupuncture Points*, Draycott Publishing, 2017; and Michael Reed Gach, *Acupressure for Lovers: Secrets of Touch for Increasing Intimacy*, New York: Bantam, 1997.

Five Elements: Kathryn Simmons Flynn, *Cooking for Fertility*, The Fertile Soul, 2010 (Kathryn is also the founder of Fertile Foods, www.fertilefoods.com); Randine Lewis, *The Infertility Cure: The Ancient Chinese Wellness*

Program for Getting Pregnant and Having Healthy Babies, New York: Little Brown, 2004 (the Fertile Soul Program includes retreats led by Randine, www.thefertilesoul.com); and Yaron Seidman, *Curing Infertility: The Incredible Hunyuan Breakthrough*, New York: Skyhorse Publishing, 2013.

Herbs and formulas for the libido. Products made by Panaxea, can be ordered at my website, www.NaturalHealingAcupuncture.com, or call 310-473-7474.

Personal products. Skin-deep database from the Environmental Working Group (www.EWG.org), dedicated to protecting health and the environment, www.ewg.org/skindeep/#.W4mwxpNKiuV; Beauty Counter is a skin-care and makeup company that has banned over 1,500 toxins from their products, www.beautycounter.com/denisewiesner.

Women's empowerment and the sacred feminine. Retreats for women that "evoke the possible," www.evokethepossible.love and www.facebook.com/everywomansvoice; and Ayurveda-informed skills and wisdom for women, www.ayurmama.com.

Women's sexual wellness, somatic healing, and yoga. Lara Catone is a social artist who teaches sex education, transformative education, and leadership training, www.laracatone.com; Hala Khouri is a trauma-certified yoga instructor who also offers somatic counseling, www.halakhouri.com; Dustienne Miller offers yoga videos for pelvic health "at your own pace," https://flourishphysicaltherapy.com/yoga-for-pelvic-health/your-pace-yoga-videos; Dr. Robin Saraswati Marcus offers "Dao Flow Yoga" for fertility and women's health, www.nourishinglife.com; Brenda Strong teaches "strong yoga for women" and offers classes, workshops, and other products, www.strongyoga4women.com; and www.yogaanytime.com; www.yogaglo.com.

CHAPTER 8. THE FIVE-ELEMENT LOVER'S WHEEL
Energy balancing. Lorie Eve Dechar, *Five Spirits: Alchemical Acupuncture for Psychological and Spiritual Healing*, New York: Lantern Books, 2006;

and Kenneth S. Cohen, *The Way of Qi Gong: The Art and Science of Chinese Energy Healing*, New York: Ballantine, 1997.

CHAPTER 9. FIRE AND FLAME

Education. Nik Douglas and Penny Slinger, *Sexual Secrets: The Alchemy of Ecstasy*, Rochester, Vt.: Destiny Books, 1979; and the American Association of Sexuality Educators, Counselors, and Therapists (AASECT), www.aasect.org/referral-directory.

Natural fertility tests. Basal body temperature charting, www.fertilityfriend.com or www.tcoyf.com/charting.aspx; and moxabustion, a traditional Chinese medicine therapy that consists of burning dried mugwort on acupuncture points on the body.

CHAPTER 10. SETTING THE STAGE

Inner guidance and feng shui. Doreen Virtue, *Goddess Guidance Oracle Cards*, Carlsbad, Ca.: Hay House, 2004; and Rodika Tchi (www.tchiconsulting.com) consults for private residences and businesses worldwide and is the feng shui expert for about.com, and she also writes for www.KnowFengShui.com.

CHAPTER 11. HEALING TRAUMA, LETTING GO OF SHAME

Books on healing trauma. Yvonne R. Farrell, *Psycho-Emotional Pain and the Eight Extraordinary Vessels*, London and Philadelphia: Singing Dragon, 2016; and Peter A. Levine, *Waking the Tiger: Healing Trauma*. Berkeley, Ca.: North Atlantic Books, 1997 (also check out Peter's website, www.somaticexperiencing.com).

Fertility practitioners offering sexual/trauma medicine. American Board of Oriental Reproductive Medicine (ABORM), aborm.org; Hazel Williams-Carter is a "traumacologist" who offers somatic attachment and trauma resolution, www.healingtraumacenter.com; and the International Society for Sexual Medicine (ISSM) offers research into sexual guidelines and health, www.issm.info.

Trauma therapies. Eye-Movement Desensitization and Reprocessing, EMDR Institute, www.emdr.com; and family constellation therapy, the Hellinger Institute of Northern California, www.hellingerpa.com.

CHAPTER 12. RELEASING STRESS

Acupuncture. How to locate the ear point Shen Men, at www.earseeds.com and at www.youtube.com/watch?v=F262_HBjZIk.

Meditation for stress reduction. Jack Kornfield, www.jackkornfield.com, is an author and Buddhist teacher who introduced mindfulness practice to the West and offers mindfulness retreats at Spirit Rock, www.spiritrock.org, a retreat center located in Woodacre, California; insight meditation teachings and retreats are listed at www.insightLA.org and www.dharmaseed.org; Tara Brach is a clinical psychologist and the founder of the Insight Meditation Community of Washington, DC (IMCW), whose website, www.tarabrach.com, offers podcasts; the Transcendental Meditation (TM) website, www.tm.org, offers complete information on this respected technique, including teachers of TM; the Living/Dying Project offers a forgiveness meditation, www.livingdying.org/forgiveness-meditation; everything you need to know about yoga nidra, including courses and teachers, is available at www.yoganidranetwork.org; and Brenda Feuerstein, a traditional hatha yoga teacher, offers a yoga nidra audio at https://soundcloud.com/traditional-yoga-studies/yoga-nidra-by-brenda-l-feuerstein.

Meditations and programs for fertility. Organic Conceptions offers a program to optimize your emotional health for conception, www.organic-conceptions.com; Circle Bloom says, "Take the stress out of trying to conceive with our free fertility meditation program," https://circlebloom.com?ref=8289; and the Seed Fertility Program, www.seedfertility.com, offers an online fertility classroom.

Mind-body work. Kundalini yoga for the "Venus kriyas" available at www.yoga/kriyas; https://www.3ho.org/.

CHAPTER 13. DEEPENING INTIMACY

Books. David Schnarch is the author of *Passionate Marriage: Keeping Love and Intimacy Alive in Committed Relationships*, New York: W.W. Norton, 1997 (and is the co-director of the Marriage and Family Health Center, crucibletherapy.com/about/david-schnarch); and Gary Chapman, *The 5 Love Languages: The Secret to Love that Lasts*, Chicago, Ill.: Northfield Publishing, 1992—and you can find out your language on his website, www.5lovelanguages.com/gary-chapman.

Education. Dawn Cartwright, tantra teacher and educator, offers workshops, www.dawncartwright.com; Emily Morse's *Sex with Emily* podcasts, blog, and products at www.sexwithemily.com; sex coach Betty Martin has the "3-minute game" on her website, www.Bettymartin.org, or go to www.sexualhealthinstitute.blogspot.com/2012/08/three-minute-game.html; and Dr. Celina Criss, sex coach and educator, offers stories, blog posts, and more at www.simplysxy.com/articles/author/celina-criss.

Video. "Look Refugees in the Eye," a powerful video that breaks down barriers, at www.amnesty.org/en/latest/news/2016/05/look-refugees-in-the-eye.

Yoga. Kiki Lovelace, yoga and pilates instructor, www.kikilovelaceyoga.com; for kirtan, a form of call-and-response chanting, check out Jai Uttal and Krishna Das.

CHAPTER 14. FOREPLAY

Books. Author and sex educator Sheri Winston, *Women's Anatomy of Arousal: Secret Maps to a Buried Treasure*, New York: Mango Garden Press (and you can find her online at https://intimateartscenter.com).

Education. Sarah Marshutz, women's empowerment workshop leader, at www.selfistry.com.

Erotica, print and video. Good sources available at www.goodreads.com, www.yourtango.com, www.amazon.com, www.goodvibes.com, www.bdsmcafe.com.

Movement and yoga. Biodanza, www.dancebiodanza.co.up/what-is-biodanza; Five Rhythms, www.5rhythms.com; ecstatic dance, www.ecstaticdance.org; and partner yoga, www.wellandgood.com/good-sweat/10-partner-yoga-poses-strengthen-relationship, and www.gaia.com/video/partner-yoga-intermediate-level?fullplayer=previe.

Sex products and adult toys. The Pleasure Chest, www.thepleasurechest.com; Adam and Eve, www.adameve.com; Jack and Jill, www.jackandjilladult.com; Good Vibrations, www.goodvibes.com; Screaming O, www.screamingo.com; Pop (maker of a strap-on dildo), www.popdildo.com; Yes Yes Yes Company, www.yesyesyes.com (certified organic); Fairhaven Health Fertility Products Babydance lubricant, https://shareasale.com/r.cfm?b=118222&u=1783625&m=16745&urllink=&afftrack=; and for everyday use, www.goodcleanlove.com; and Sunny Rogers, a certified sex coach and clinical sexologist, is the brand manager and sexual health educator for three top intimate products manufacturers, Pipedream Products, Jimmyjane, and Sir Richard's, www.coachsunnyrodgers.com.

CHAPTER 15. THE BIG O

Books. Lai Hsi, *The Sexual Teachings of the White Tigress: Secrets of the Female Taoist Masters*, Rochester, Vt.: Destiny Books, 2001.

Eco-sexuality. Find out more about "Earth as lover" at www.theecosexuals.ucsc.edu.

Education. Interactive website on sexuality where real people share their intimate sexual stories, www.OMGYES.com.

Get off antidepressants (SSRIs) naturally. Dr. Hyla Cass, "A New Vision of Health Care," www.cassmd.com.

CHAPTER 16. WHEN YOU NEED A HAND

Erectile dysfunction. Dr. Kathryn Retzler's podcast at www.webmd.com/erectile-dysfunction/guide/drugs-linked-erectile-dysfunction.

Libido issues. Mayo Clinic on low sex drive for men and women, www.mayoclinic.org.

O and P shot. Robyn Benson, http://robynbenson.com.

Pelvic pain. Physical therapist Deena Poll Goodman specializes in pelvic pain, www.goodmanphysicaltherapy.com.

Pelvic-floor DVDs. Physical therapist and yoga therapist Dustienne Miller offers pelvic-pain videos that integrate yoga with pelvic-floor exercises, www.yourpaceyoga.com.

Index

About the Author

DENISE WIESNER LAC., DIPL. AC., founder of the Natural Healing & Acupuncture Clinic in West Los Angeles, is an internationally recognized traditional Chinese medicine practitioner, specializing in the Whole Systems Chinese medicine approach to women's health, sexuality, and fertility. Since 1994, Denise has treated and helped women manage challenges from menstrual disorders through menopause and from infertility to pregnancy. Using a combination of acupuncture, diet and lifestyle counseling, nutritional supplements, and Chinese herbs, Denise has helped thousands of couples navigate the tricky, and often stressful, journey toward fertility, without losing their loving connection.

She has a BA in exercise kinesiology (UCLA), an MA in traditional Chinese medicine (Emperor's College), and is a certified sex coach. She is board-certified by the State of California and the American Board of Oriental Reproductive Medicine (ABORM), and a charter member of the Fertile Soul: Clinical Excellence in Fertility program.

Denise teaches professional seminars to medical doctors, ob-gyns, and nurse midwives on the application of Chinese medicine in obstetrics and gynecology and has published articles on acupuncture and infertility. In addition to a thriving private practice, Denise lectures at conferences, works closely with reproductive endocrinologists, and is a professor in the doctoral program in Chinese Medicine, Fertility, and Women's Health at Yo San University.

In her spare time, she relishes practicing yoga, playing guitar, dancing, and hanging out with her two sons, Noah and Ethan.